NUTRITION and HEALTH

Fighting Diabetes, Cancer & Heart Disease

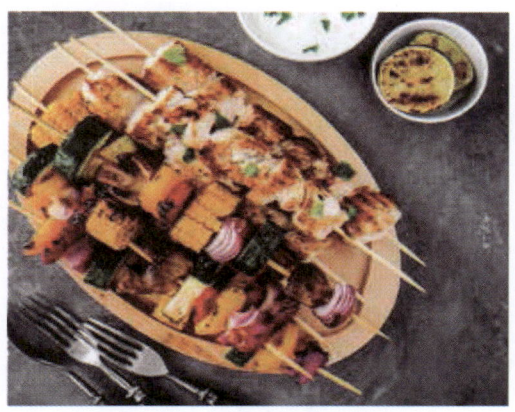

The power of Super Nutrients in Reversing Chronic Diseases
Weight Loss Tips and Sample Menus

Rosemary Wachira RD CDCES

Copyright © 2021 Rosemary Wachira RD CDCES
All rights reserved
First Edition

PAGE PUBLISHING, INC.
Conneaut Lake, PA

First originally published by Page Publishing 2021

ISBN 978-1-64701-925-9 (pbk)
ISBN 978-1-64701-926-6 (digital)

Printed in the United States of America

CONTENTS

Introduction 5

1. Change in Diet Trends: From Cultural to Urban and Modern City Diets 9
2. Preventing and Controlling Diabetes Through Healthy Diets 27
3. Cancer Preventive and Cancer-Fighting Nutrition 47
4. Heart Health: Foods to Lower Blood Pressure and Blood Cholesterol 70
5. Losing Weight and Keeping It Off 83
6. Lifestyle Change & Sample Menus For Diabetes, Cancer, Heart Disease, & Weight Loss 96
7. The Healing Kitchen: Using Superfoods to Fight Chronic Diseases 116

INTRODUCTION

Food and Health

Health benefits obtained from healthy diets and the healing properties found in plant foods have been researched by many doctors and scientists and proven to be supreme in prevention of chronic illnesses. The use of food in healing and in disease prevention goes way back in time to the days of the famous Greek philosopher Hippocrates, who is referred to as the father of medicine. Hippocrates made the famous statement "Let food be your medicine, and let medicine be your food." This statement has been widely used by modern-day doctors, by nutritionists, and other health-care professionals as book titles and in health education articles.

The concept of using food as medicine has gained increasing interest and is well accepted in many parts of the world. There are numerous research studies supporting the role of foods in disease prevention, many studies indicating that plant foods contain more than macro nutrients, vitamins and minerals, but also contain powerful molecules known to have positive effects in prevention of chronic illnesses. Plant foods containing proven healing nutrients are referred to as "super foods."

Most people who were raised in rural areas or in farmlands, whether in African countries, Asian countries, the Caribbean islands, or in South America, have seen either grandparents or parents use different plants, roots, and herbs as home remedies. My parents and grandparent would use aloe vera leaves fresh from the farm to treat skin cuts or abrasions as a way to prevent infection. They also kept honey harvested from their beehives and used it as remedies for coughs and common colds and many other home remedies.

This book discusses the changes in diet trends as people moved from farmlands to urban towns and cities. It compares cultural or old ways diets that were mainly plant-based foods that provided adequate amounts of proteins, vitamins, minerals, macronutrients, and phytonutrients. These foods contained high amounts of fiber and small amounts of cholesterol-free fats compared to the new urban city diets that are high in processed foods, high in fat, cholesterol, and sodium but low in fiber, vitamins, minerals, and phytonutrients. This book also shows how diet changes to the "Western-style diets," such as fried foods, fast-food meals, and high-fat breakfast foods correlates to an increase in chronic diseases, such as diabetes, hypertension, cancer, heart disease, etc. commonly seen in Western countries but, in recent years, have increased at alarming rates in sub-Saharan Africa and in other developing countries.

Each chapter in this book digs more into the word health benefits of reducing high-fat foods, highly processed foods, and replacing them with healthy whole plant foods that allow body detoxing, replenishing of body cells and organs, and reducing body inflammation. This book also discusses how increasing or including foods containing healing properties helps reverse diseases such as high blood sugar, blood cholesterol, blood pressure, and help reverse other chronic illnesses. Based on food science research on health benefits of plant foods, I agree with the Greek philosopher's statement on using food as medicine as we see chronic diseases being reversed through healthy diets and healthy lifestyles.

CHAPTER 1

Change in Diet Trends: From Cultural to Urban and Modern City Diets

For many generations, our ancestors consumed farm fresh foods which included whole grains such as corn/maize, millet, sorghum, and a variety of beans. The diets also included a variety of beans and bananas, starchy tubers, such as sweet potatoes, cassava, arrow roots and yams plus different varieties of fresh leafy greens. These traditional foods were cultivated using only natural fertilizers from plants and animal dung. The foods contained no chemicals or conventional pesticides which are used in large-scale farming in many countries. In our modern-day cities, such foods are referred to in supermarkets as "organic foods" and are sold at a higher cost than foods grown using chemicals, bioengineered or genetically modified foods, and processed foods. In other words, our ancestors consumed only organic foods.

Whole Grains and Seeds

A review of different ancestral meals shows that most cultural foods included whole grains as part of their main meals. A whole grain food contains all three parts of the seed[1] as indicated below: The germ, which is the smallest yellowish part of the seed has the potential to germinate into a sprout or plant and is sometimes referred to as the embryo or the life of the seed. The germ contains the important mineral iron which is needed for healthy blood. It contains vitamin E, an essential vitamin for healthy body cells and plays important role in building a strong immune system. The germ also contains vitamins and minerals and small amounts of healthy fats.

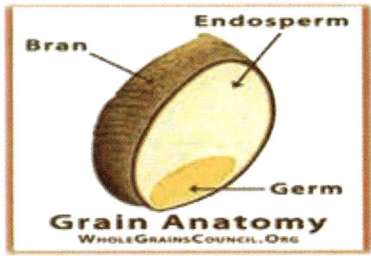

The endosperm is the middle layer of the seed. It usually contains complex carbohydrates and is a good source of energy in a meal. The endosperm also contains some protein and B vitamins. The third part of a seed is bran which is the outer shell of the grain or seed. Bran is high in fiber and several important B vitamins such as folate, thiamine, and niacin. Research shows that consumption of bran in whole grains promotes healthy bowel functions and has been proven to reduce consti-

---

[1] Oldways Whole Grain Council, https://wholegrainscouncil.org/whole-grains-101/health. Photo by Whole Grain Council.

pation and diseases of the colon, such as diverticulosis and colorectal cances.[2]

Consuming whole grains provides the body with a much higher nutrient content than processed grains. Whole grains are not only high in fiber, vitamins, and minerals but also much higher in naturally occurring phytonutrients. The refining process removes two important parts of the grain: bran and germ. Removing these two parts of the grain results in the loss of fiber, important B vitamins, vitamin E, iron, and healthy fats found in the germ. Additionally, processed grains lose important disease-fighting phytonutrients known to prevent chronic illnesses[3]. Depriving the body of these various powerful vitamins, minerals, and phytonutrients increases the risk of chronic illnesses.

Refined grains are milled and processed to yield soft textured products such as white bread, pastries, cookies, cakes, mandazis, soft-textured ugali, white rice, and other products. Table 1 shows disease-fighting power available in whole grains. The recommended intake of whole grains such as brown rice, whole wheat, sorghum, millet, and oats is 3–4 servings daily. Examples of a servings

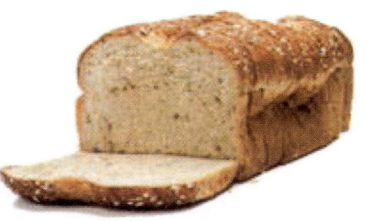

Credit to Whole Grain Council

---

[2] World Cancer Research Fund, American Institute of Cancer Research, "Diet, Nutrition, Physical Activity and Cancer: A Global Perspective—Continuous Update Project Expert Report," 54–55.

[3] Sharon Rady Rolfes, Kathryn Pinna, and Ellie Whitney, *Understanding Normal and Clinical Nutrition 7th Edition*, 161.

is one sliced bread, one and a half cup oatmeal, etc. For more details on serving sizes, see table 2B.

Table 1A. Nutrients in Whole grains[*4]	
Vitamins and Minerals	**Key Functions**
B Vitamins: niacin, riboflavin, and thiamin,	<ul><li>Good for metabolism. B vitamins help release energy from protein, carbohydrates, and fats.</li><li>Essential for healthy nervous system.</li></ul>
Iron	<ul><li>Iron transports oxygen in red blood cells. Good sources are beans and lentils.</li></ul>
Folate (Folic Acid)	<ul><li>Helps the body form red blood cells.</li><li>Prevents neural tube birth defects during fetal development.</li></ul>
Vitamin E	<ul><li>Vitamin E is an antioxidant, prevents cell damage from free radicals, and helps the body's immune system stay strong.</li></ul>
Phosphorus and Magnesium	<ul><li>Phosphorus works with calcium to help form strong healthy bones and teeth.</li><li>Magnesium helps with important transmission of nerve signals in the body.</li></ul>

---

[4] Table 1, https://wholegrainscouncil.org/blog/2016/06/whole-grain-value-2-3-times-more-most nutrients.

Potassium	<ul><li>Potassium is one of the major electrolytes in the blood. It helps maintains fluid and electrolyte balance.</li><li>Muscle contraction and normal nerve transmission.</li></ul>
Calcium	<ul><li>Calcium supports strong bones and teeth.</li><li>It plays an important role in healthy muscle contraction and normal nerve functions.</li></ul>
Zinc	<ul><li>It supports healthy immune system.</li><li>Healthy body cell division for growth and development and proper wound healing.</li><li>Taste and smell perception.</li><li>Helps in metabolism of carbohydrates.</li></ul>

Common Ethnic Foods

In many cultures, staple foods included a variety of bean and maize meals that are still used today in many countries. The variety of beans used included black beans, red kidney beans, pigeon peas, chickpeas, pinto beans and white-eyed beans, called njaji beans in Kenya, mung beans, etc. were used to create tasty ethnic meals. Most cultures used maize and beans combination as the main meals. This meal has remained popular among many cultures. A popular dish in Kenya, maize and bean dish, commonly referred to as Githeri, is basically boiled beans and maize with a pinch of salt. Githeri is commonly served with no added fat; however, adding or topping a plate of githeri with an avocado adds loads of vitamins and minerals, healthy fats, and adds great taste to the dish. In some cultures, the top layer/bran of maize is removed to make a soft textured meal called muthokoi, which is lower in fiber than githeri. Kenyan cultural meals also include maize and beans with added potatoes, bananas, and leafy greens mashed together to make another popular dish referred to as "Mukimo." Mukimo dishes come in different varieties depending on the type of beans and the type of leafy greens used in the recipes. The meals could be made with kidney beans, pigeon peas or njugu beans, pinto beans, green peas, etc. Many cultures use greens that are available in different seasons and could range from pumpkin leaves, cassava leaves, stinging nettles, and many other varieties of leafy greens.

Maize and beans meals are commonly used for all three meals in many African countries. The difference in our modern-day cooking from the cultural meals is the improved recipes, by adding either other ingredients, oil, spices and flavors as preferred in different cultures. An example would be South African tasty chakalaka bean stew made with vegetables and spices. The stew makes a great meal for lunch or dinner meals. West Africans make bean puddings called Moimoi that are great with lunch or dinner. Coconut bean meals are more popular in coastal regions. Pigeon beans with coconut or Bahaazi beans are common breakfast meals in East African coastal regions.

Bean Nutrition

Beans have been declared by the World Health Organization (WHO) and the American Academy of Nutrition as miracle foods due to their high nutrient content, affordability, and multiple health benefits. Beans are good sources protein, carbohydrates, and fiber, plus several phytochemicals and antioxidants. A cup of beans provides between 9-13 grams of protein, depending on the type of beans used, making beans a healthy plant protein which can replace high fat, high cholesterol meats or animal proteins for the heart-healthy individual or those with high blood cholesterol levels. Beans are not only good sources of protein and carbohydrates but also provides several B vitamins, folate, and iron. The iron in beans is the non-heme iron found in plant foods and is more easily absorbed in the body than the heme iron found in meats.[5] Iron is an essential mineral needed in red blood cells in transport of oxygen from the lungs to all body tissues. Beans are 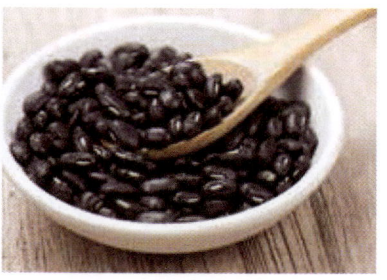 also a good source of calcium, the mineral that helps build and maintain healthy bones and teeth, and they are also good sources of potassium and magnesium. Beans, peas, and lentils are great sources of soluble and insoluble fibers. Soluble fiber in beans helps protect

---

[5] Janet Bond Brill, *Cholesterol Down*, 114.

against heart disease by lowering LDL/low-density lipoproteins or bad cholesterol in the blood, preventing plaque-like cholesterol buildup in blood vessels, making beans heart healthy food.[6]

- The combination of carbohydrates, protein, and high fiber in beans makes beans low glycemic index food due to the slowed release of glucose in the gut following digestion. Glycemic index is used as a measure of how quickly a consumed food causes blood sugar to rise or increase. The measure ranks glycemic index of foods from a range of 1–100. Foods with a glycemic index range of 0–55 are considered low glycemic index foods. Beans and lentils range from 29–39 on the Glycemic Index charts and are low glycemic foods.[7]
- All bean varieties including kidney beans, black beans, pinto beans, and lentils are high in antioxidants and phytonutrients, naturally occurring molecules in plant foods that are known to help the body fight against cancer (see chapter 3 on cancer nutrition).

---

[6] Bond Brill, 115.
[7] Neal Barnard, *Dr. Neal Barnard's Program for Reversing Diabetes. The Scientifically Proven System for Reversing Diabetes without Drugs*, 56.

Other Staple Foods

Beans and lentils were used as main protein foods in many cultures. Root vegetables were the main source of carbohydrates and a great source of energy. Meats were not a common part of daily diet but were used on occasions. Farm animals were slaughtered during important family events and celebrations, such as youth coming-of-age celebrations, birth of a child: during marriage ceremonies. Other sources of protein included fresh fish available to people who lived near large bodies of water. People who lived in Africa's coastal regions and those who lived near freshwater lakes, or large rivers, enjoyed a variety of fresh fish all year round. East Africans who currently reside in coastal regions, or near large rivers and large bodies of water such as Lake Turkana and Lake Victoria regions consume a variety of nutritious fish all year. A common dish for people residing around Lake Victoria region is the omena fish, referred to as *dagaa* by people of Tanzania and *mukene* in Uganda. The fish is cooked and consumed whole from head to tail and is a great source of protein, iron, and omega-3 heart healthy fats similar to other fatty fish such as salmon, smelt, and sardines, etc.

Cultural Breakfast Choices

Breakfast foods in most cultural diets included a bowl of hot cereal made from millet and sorghum or maize. Other breakfast food included either boiled or fire roasted: Cassava, sweet potatoes, yams, plantains/bananas, and arrowroots. They also consumed tender farm fresh, fire grilled or steamed maize cobs, or leftover maize and bean mix (githeri).

Cereal Grains

One of the most common breakfast cereals is hot millet cereal referred to as uji ya wimbi in East African countries. Uji is made from a combination of millet, sorghum, and maize flour or just millet and maize flour. The original sour uji was made by mixing millet and maize flour and water and allowing the pasty mixture to sit and ferment in natural gourds for about 2-3 days before cooking to give it a flavorful tangy taste. In our modern-day kitchens, a quick shortcut to the fermentation process is adding lemon juice to fresh cooked millet porridge, which gives it a similar flavor, but less gut probiotics than those in naturally fermented porridge. Millet cereal/uji is served as hot cereal in the morning and as a cold afternoon beverage during hot sunny days. This sweet, flavorful hot breakfast cereal provides important vitamins, minerals, and phytonutrients. Health benefits of grains such as millet and sorghum are impressive. Millet is a good source of B vitamins, good source of calcium, magnesium, and phosphorus, it's a good source of fiber and it is a gluten-free cereal for those who suffer from gluten intolerance. Both sorghum and millet help lower LDL or bad cholesterol in the body, and they contain phytonutrients and antioxidants that are powerful in fighting chronic illnesses including cancer.[8]

---

[8] Taste of African Heritage by Oldways, https://wholegrainscouncil.org/whole-grains-101/whole-grains-101-orphan-pages-found/

The largest producers of millet in Africa include Nigeria, Niger, Ethiopia and Tanzania but millet is grown and used in most African countries. Millet and sorghum are highly popular in East African countries not only as breakfast food but also commonly used to make millet ugali, a more nutritious side dish made with maize floor and millet similar in consistency to South African pap, phaleche and West African fufu. Millet is used in injera bread recipes by people of Ethiopia. In Nigeria millet is used to make the popular breakfast spicy fermented porridge. My friends tell me that in Zimbabwe and Southern Africa millet is used to make a tasty side dish called sadza, and in India and part of Pakistan, millet flour is often added to chapati and roti recipes.

Healthy Snacks

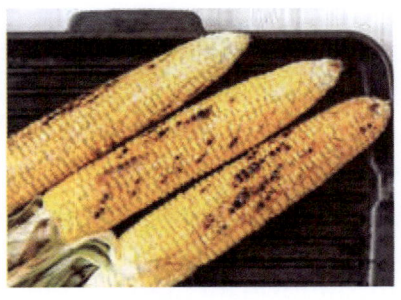

Foods consumed as snacks especially on days that families worked long hours in their farms included a variety of sun-ripe seasonal fruits such as mangos, papayas, ripe bananas, passion fruits, avocados, a variety of black and red berries, golden berries and other mulberries, sugarcanes, honey from farmed beehives, nuts, etc. Beverages used for late afternoon snacks for those looking after cattle or those who

---

health-benefits-millet.

worked long hours in the farms included kefir, kefir/ *maziwa-lala*, a high protein beverage and a favorite meal among Kalenjin, Masai, Kisii of Kenya, and other nomadic cultures in Southern and Western parts of Africa. Another common beverage was fermented porridge, which was kept cool in dry gourd vessels to be used by farmers as needed. These beverages were packed with protein, carbohydrates, water, and electrolytes such as potassium and sodium great for replenishment on hot sunny days.

These meals and snacks provided the macro nutrients listed below, plus a load of vitamins, minerals, fiber and powerful phytonutrients:

1. Carbohydrates from starchy foods such as maize/corn and root vegetables such as potatoes, yams, sweet potatoes, cassava, green bananas, millet, sorghum, and also from fresh fruits.
2. Protein sources include beans and lentils, nuts, small amounts of milk, and kefir.
3. Fats: Whole grains and beans contain minimal amounts of healthy fats needed for meal satisfaction and to provide fat soluble vitamins in the body.
4. Vitamins, minerals, antioxidants and phytonutrients from whole grains, beans, leafy greens, nuts and fruits.

Honey: Sweetener and Natural medicine

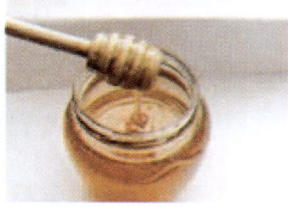

Honey and bee-hive products such as bee pollen, propolis and royal jelly are considered superfoods due to their high nutrient contents, and powerful antibiotic properties. When consumed in its original raw unprocessed state, honey and bee pollen are loaded with antioxidants and healing nutrients. Our ancestors harvested and ate honey combs containing all the bee-hive products with meals and snacks. Honey contains digestive enzymes great for irritable bowels and other gastrointestinal problems. Bee pollen is considered a complete food as it contains carbohydrates, protein and amino acids, several B vitamins, Vitamins C, D and E, calcium, potassium phosphorous, iron and other microminerals.[9] Honey and Pollen are used to treat the common cough and cold, also used for treatments of common seasonal allergies.

Changing Trends to City Diets and Lifestyles

Like many other developing nations across the globe, as people move from countryside to the cities and urban towns in search of employment, the trend in diets also changed to the more available urban meals and quick cooking foods. Likewise, in modern-day cities in sub-Saharan African countries, people who were raised

---

[9] *Wolf David. The Food and Medicine of the Future page 87.*

on indigenous low-fat plant-based diets full of whole grains, beans, healthy root tubers, and vegetables were introduced to high-fat, low-fiber city meals, including processed white breads with butter, white flour pastries, mandazis, chapatis for breakfast, high-fat fried potatoes, and sausages for lunch. Economic status or affordability of certain foods and beverages plays a big role in foods and snacks consumed. For most people in urban living, their meals increased in processed foods, mixed with some days of ethnic meals as available. Dinner meals, which are mostly consumed at home, contains more vegetables and whole grains than breakfast and lunch meals which are consumed during morning rash hours or during the work day. The table below compares some common city meals to country cooking among the people of Kenya.

Table 1B. Cultural vs. Modern-Day Meals

Cultural Style Breakfast and Lunch Meals	City Breakfast and Lunch Meals
A bowl of whole grain cereal or porridge made with millet and sorghum or whole maize flour, boiled sweet potatoes, or fire-roasted maize	Tea with milk and sugar, white bread, mandazis, coffee cake and pastries, fried eggs, sausage, and bacon, pancake with syrup or donuts

Lunch Meals

Mixed maize and bean githeri, muthokoi with lentils, pumpkins, sweet potatoes, banana meals, coconut beans, mukimo with greens, kefir/maziwa lala. Millet ugali or whole grain maize ugali with large servings of leafy greens, fresh fruits as desired, small amounts of fresh fish for those who dwelled around large bodies of water	Low cost lunch meal: chips/french fries, half a loaf of bread with soda or tea, chicken with chips, or samosa with tea. Restaurant meals: grilled beef or goat meats/choma, chicken, hamburger, fried potatoes, white rice, small amounts of vegetables, sodas, and beers
Benefits: Whole grain nutrients, low fat, low cholesterol, low sodium, and high in fiber, good for heart health. High in cancer-fighting nutrients and high in nutrients that help control blood pressure. Foods with low GI index helpful for blood sugar control	*These foods are high in calories, high in cholesterol and salt/sodium, but low in fiber and important disease fighting nutrients. Refined grain foods have a higher glycemic index and ccontributes to high blood sugar levels in the body.*

Diet and Disease Prevention

Urban living has not only affected our food and beverage choices but has added new social events, such as afterwork evening get-togethers, movies, or outings, where people may consume high-fat snacks or meals, soft drinks high in sugar, and for some people, alcoholic beverages. High-fat restaurant meals or fried meats and high-fat fast foods including pizza, high sugar beverages, and alcoholic drinks adds extra calories and carbohydrates to the daily intake. Consuming low-fiber high calorie meals that are high in fat and cholesterol, high in sugar, and high in sodium contributes to excess weight gain, obesity, and increases the risk of chronic illnesses such as high-blood pressure, diabetes, heart disease, and cancer.[10] These chronic illnesses were not common in the old country lifestyles but are now increasingly common not only among those living in cities and urban areas, but also among those living in the countrysides but regularly consume processed foods. Some farmers sell farm produce and use their earned income to purchase less healthy processed foods such as white bread, white rice, sugar, soda, cupcakes, cookies, etc.

The commonly used phrases such as "prevention is better than cure, or the phrase "an ounce of prevention is better than a pound of cure" all comes to mind when we see the devastation brought on by preventable chronic illnesses such as diabetes, hypertension, cancer, and heart

---

[10] T. Colin Campbell and Thomas Campbell II, *The China Study: Revised and Expanded Edition*, 66.

disease. These chronic illnesses can be easily prevented, treated, or reversed through healthy diets and healthy lifestyles. Meals high in plant foods, such as beans, vegetables, grains, nuts, and fruits contain antioxidants and phytonutrients, proven to be highly effective in fighting chronic illnesses. Healthy diets should include a variety of beans and lentils, a variety of vegetables and whole grains as part of diet. Beans and lentils provide adequate amounts of healthy protein comparable to that in meats but without the high fat and high cholesterol found in meats. Cholesterol is a major cause of clogged arteries and heart disease. Consider reducing red meats, high-fat pork, and processed meats that are high in cholesterol and sodium, such as breakfast sausage links and dinner sausages, bacon, hot dogs, and other high cholesterol foods. Choose white meats, such as fish, chicken, turkey. Include healthy complex carbohydrates, such as maize, green bananas, potatoes and sweet potato, yams cassava, and other root vegetables.

> Phytonutrients: Special compounds found in plant foods that help the body fight and prevent various illnesses.

Beverages contribute to total calories and carbohydrate contents in meals. Sugar sweetened beverages such as soda, fruit punch, sports drinks, flavored coffees, flavored teas etc. contains high amounts of sugar. Soda contains about 10 teaspoons in small cans and about 16 teaspoons in the larger 16-ounce soda bottles. Consuming these high sugar beverages increases total carbohydrates intake in a meal. Consuming high-sugar beverages and high-sugar snacks, such as cookies, cakes, donuts, and candy bars adds extra calories in the diet, leading to unwanted weight gain, obesity, and increased risk of type 2 diabetes. Choose healthy low-fat, low-sugar snacks, such as fresh fruits. Choose low-sugar beverages, such as herbal tea, green tea, millet porridge, chai tea, and adequate amounts of water.

Living in modern cities means less access or availability of farm-fresh produce for most people. However, supermarkets and grocery stores sell a variety of seasonally available fresh vegetables and fruits. Some grocery stores provide fresh fruits and vegetables from the local farmers. Most supermarkets also sell frozen vegetables that could be used whenever fresh vegetables are out of season. While we may not have access to garden fresh or farm to table foods, we have access to whole grains, a variety of beans, vegetables, and fruits all year long. Consuming whole plants foods provides the body with adequate protein, complex carbohydrates, vitamins and minerals, and super nutrients needed to fight and prevent chronic illnesses.

CHAPTER 2

Preventing and Controlling Diabetes Through Healthy Diets

Diabetes is a chronic disease caused by blood sugar levels that are higher than normal. High blood sugars occur when the pancreas is no longer able to make adequate amounts of insulin or when the body is unable to make use of the insulin available in the body leading to elevated blood sugars or diabetes. According to the World Health Organization report, type 2 diabetes has increased at an alarming rate in Kenya and many African countries in the last ten to twenty years.[11] There are many people who have diabetes and may not know they have it, others might be mistaking symptoms of diabetes as just being tired and fatigued from work. Most people find out they have diabetes while seeking medical treatment as the symptoms persist.

---

[11] https://www.who.int/features/2014/kenya-rising-diabetes/en/.

Symptoms of Diabetes

Diabetes causes a high concentration of blood sugar or glucose in the bloodstream, but at the same time there is a shortage of blood glucose in cells and muscles. Since blood sugar / glucose is the main source of energy in muscles and body organs such as heart and brain, the inadequate supply of glucose causes a feeling of fatigue and tiredness even after hours of rest. Some people may not experience any symptoms, others might experience a few symptoms while others may experience most of the symptoms listed below.[12]

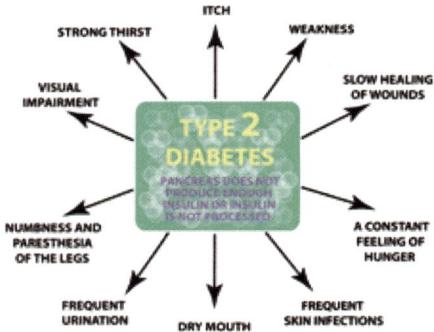

- tiredness and fatigue
- unquenchable thirst
- frequent urination.
- undesired weight loss
- extreme hunger
- blurry vision

---

[12] Barnard, 4.

Frequent Thirst and Frequent Urination

It's common for people with high blood sugars or undiagnosed diabetes to experience insatiable thirst. They could drink large cups of water, juice, soda, or other beverages in an attempt to quench their thirst, but no matter what they drink or how much they drink still feel thirsty within a few minutes. Drinking soda and high sugar beverages such as punch and sweet tea or fruit juices causes the blood sugar buildup to rise even higher. The more liquids the individual drinks, the more frequent the urge to urinate, creating a cycle of drinking and running to the toilet/bathroom.

Weight Loss

People with undiagnosed diabetes may experience undesired or unplanned weight loss even though they have not changed their diet, and are eating same types of foods and same portions as usual. Having diabetes or high blood sugar in blood vessels means that the blood glucose or energy from foods consumed is not being delivered to the cells in muscles and organs where it's needed, causing the individual to experience hunger within a short time after eating a meal. While blood sugar remains high, the starving cells are continuously sending signals to the brain that they need glucose or energy. The body finds an alternative source of energy, usually from body fat stores. When the stored fat is broken down and used to provide the energy required by vital organs such as heart and brain, it causes unplanned weight loss. Inadequate insulin in the body and continuously high blood sugar levels could cause dehydration, nausea, vomiting and could lead to a dangerous condition known as diabetic ketoacidosis.

> Ketone: Formed when the body breaks down fats for energy.
> Acidosis: Caused by high ketone build up in the blood.

Blurry Vision

High levels of blood sugar inside the eye causes the eye lenses to swell, which leads to a loss of sharpness of vision. This results in temporally blurred vision; however, this is resolved once the blood sugar levels are normalized.[13]

Prediabetes

Prediabetes is a condition in which the blood sugar is slightly elevated above normal but not high enough to be diagnosed as type 2 diabetes. Having prediabetes is a sign that the insulin is not functioning at full capacity. This condition does not have symptoms, and most people find out about their slightly elevated blood sugar through a blood test. Prediabetes can be reversed through healthy diet and regular physical activity. Taking action and making lifestyle changes results in reversing blood sugars to

---

[13] Rolfes, Pinna, and Whitney, 792.

healthy levels but ignoring prediabetes could lead to type 2 diabetes.

Different Types of Diabetes

There are three main types of diabetes. Type 1 diabetes, which is rare, type 2 diabetes, which is the most common type of diabetes, and gestational diabetes, which is seen during pregnancy. Gestational diabetes is caused by increased levels of pregnancy hormones, which results in increased insulin resistance and increased insulin needs during pregnancy. General diet guidelines for gestational diabetes include adequate intake of nutrients with moderate amounts of carbohydrate foods. It's important to distribute carbohydrate foods throughout the day, preferably moderate portions in three meals, and two to three snacks, or as instructed by a medical doctor. Include whole grains, vegetables, beans, legumes, nuts, milk, yogurt, and fruits. Avoid sugar-added foods and beverages, such as soda, cakes, and pastries. Drink ginger tea for nausea avoid ginger ale sodas. See food list on table 2B. Gestational diabetes usually resolves after the baby is born, and the mom's blood sugars usually return to normal after delivery. However, women who have had gestational diabetes are at higher risk of developing type 2 diabetes later in life and need to make healthy food choices and exercise regularly to prevent type 2 diabetes.[14]

---

[14] Barnard, 8.

Type 1 Diabetes

Type 1 diabetes, also called insulin-dependent diabetes is mostly seen in young children and some youth. In type 1 diabetes, the pancreas is dysfunctional and does not produce insulin. This happens when the insulin-producing cells in the pancreas are mistakenly attacked and destroyed by the body's own immune system. The immune system normally protects the body against viruses and bacteria, but in this case, the white blood cells attack and destroy insulin-producing cells known as beta cells. The progressive destruction of beta cells leaves the pancreas unable to make insulin, resulting in high blood sugars levels or hyperglycemia. Without production of this vital hormone, people with type 1 diabetes require daily insulin injections. That's why this type of diabetes is referred to as insulin-dependent diabetes.[15]

Type 2 Diabetes

Type 2 diabetes was previously referred to as "adult-onset diabetes" and was generally seen in adult populations. However, in recent years, this type of diabetes is increasingly being diagnosed in teenagers and young adults. Type 2 diabetes is the most common type of diabetes in the world. Type 2 diabetes results from either inadequate insulin production in the pancreas, or the body cells are no longer utilizing the available insu-

---

[15] Barnard, 6.

lin correctly, which is referred to as insulin resistance. Major contributors of insulin resistance are physical inactivity, obesity, and increased fat around the stomach and internal organs which interferes with normal insulin functions. The fat accumulation in cells can be reversed through healthy diets, exercise, and weight loss.[16] According to Center for Disease Control (CDC), reducing body weight by 5–7% results in improved insulin usage and improved blood sugar levels.[17]

How Insulin Works

Following consumption of a meal, foods containing carbohydrates are digested and broken down into glucose, commonly called blood sugar. Insulin helps move the blood sugar into cells and muscles where it's used for energy or stored for later use. Since insulin is required for this vital role, inadequate production of insulin or the body's inability to utilize the available insulin leads to diabetes or high levels of blood sugar buildup in blood vessels. Insulin not only helps move and use blood sugar in the body but also affects how the body uses fats and protein from foods. It allows storage of fat and helps make protein available for use as needed in the body.[18]

The body's inability to utilize available insulin also called insulin resistance, is common in type 2 diabetes.

---

[16] Barnard, 24.

[17] http://www.diabetes.org/diabetes-basics/type-2/facts-about-type-2.html?loc=db-slabnav.

[18] Constance Brown-Riggs and Tamara Jeffries, *Living Well with Diabetes*, 16.

The pancreas produces adequate amounts of insulin, but the cells are not opening up to receive the glucose, causing blood sugar build up in blood vessels.[19] A good example of this function would be that of a lock and key. The key fits in the keyhole to unlock the door. In this example, the keyhole would be the insulin receptor on a body cell. If the keyhole is blocked, the key or insulin does not fit in to open the cells, leading to high blood sugar in the blood or diabetes.

Another cause of high blood sugar is sluggish or damaged beta cells. High insulin demands cause beta cells of the pancreas to overwork in an effort to meet high insulin requirements. The over worked beta cells get exhausted or damaged leading to reduced insulin production. Inadequate insulin in the body leads to diabetes.[20]

> *Insulin—vital hormone produced in the pancreas*
> *Insulin resistance: In insulin resistance, the body makes enough insulin, but the cells are unable to use it properly. It has been attributed to obesity and excess body fat especially around the gut or waistline. Insulin resistance is also seen with severe illness and chronic body inflammation.*

Both inadequate insulin production and insulin resistance causes the blood sugar to raise to abnormally high levels. When blood sugar remains consistently high in blood vessels, it causes an imbalance in the body that

---

[19] Kedar N. Prasad, *Fight Diabetes with Vitamins and Minerals*, 12.
[20] Prasad, 12.

causes damage to blood vessels and nerves. Poorly controlled diabetes or consistently high levels of blood glucose leads to health problems such as heart disease, eye nerve damage and blindness, stroke, kidney disease, severe kidney damage leading to need for dialysis, and damages to nerves in body extremities leading to amputations.

Diagnostic Tests for Diabetes

The most commonly used types of blood sugar tests include a fasting blood sugar test which is taken after 8 hours fast or overnight fast, and random glucose test which is completed without regard of food intake. This test is commonly used for people who have symptoms of diabetes. Hemoglobin A1c is the test that provides a history of the average blood glucose levels over the past two to three months. This test analyzes blood glucose that attaches or sticks to hemoglobin on red blood cells over a duration of two to three months. The higher the blood glucose, the higher the A1c. Fasting is not required for the A1c test.

Table 2A. Diagnostic Readings[21]

Readings	Normal	Prediabetes	Diabetes
Fasting (MG/DL)	70–99	100–125	126 or higher
Hemoglobin A1C %	Below 5.7%	5.7–6.4%	6.5 or higher

---

[21] https://www.cdc.gov/diabetes/basics/getting-tested.html.

Reversing Blood Sugars through Lifestyle Change

The first step in lowering or reversing high blood sugar is a healthy diet and regular physical activity. A healthy diet should include foods that are low in fat, low in sugar, and high in fiber. Plant foods, such as beans, lentils, vegetables, and whole grains, are usually low in fat and high in fiber. A healthy diet combined with regular physical activity helps burn off the fat, cleans out the cells, and allows normal cell functions that reverses insulin resistance and promotes normal insulin usage and improved blood sugar levels. [22]

Recommendations for healthy diets include whole grain foods, such as millet, brown rice, whole wheat bread/brown bread, whole wheat chapatis, and whole grain cereals, and corn/maize. Whole grains are high in fiber and the mineral chromium, an essential mineral that plays an important role in carbohydrate metabolism by enhancing activity of insulin.[23] High fiber foods provide a feeling of fullness that reduces eating more food than essentially needed. Other health benefits of whole grains and legumes includes slowing down absorption of glucose in the gut which helps regulate blood sugar.[24] Limit processed foods, such as white breads, white rice, pasta, noodles, pastries, cookies, cakes, and other white flour products. Include lean meats and a variety of veg-

---

[22] Barnard, 26.
[23] Rolfes, Pinna, and Whitney, 456.
[24] Rolfes, Pinna, and Whitney, 124.

etables, such as cabbages, collards, green beans, spinach, broccoli, peppers, leafy greens, etc. Vegetables are commonly served as small portions of side dishes; however, the recommended amount is 1/2 plate of cooked vegetables with lunch and dinner.

Fresh fruits are great sources of vitamins, minerals, and fiber. They make delicious low-calorie snacks between meals and a great dessert after meals; however, they are also naturally high in the sugar fructose, which is a carbohydrate. People with diabetes should consume fruit juices in moderation as juice is more concentrated and higher in carbohydrate content than fresh fruit. A glass of juice 8 fld oz contains an equivalent of two medium-sized fruits. Recommended intake of fruits is about three to four servings a day for adults. Choose fresh fruit more often than canned fruits. When purchasing canned fruit or fruit cups, choose fruits canned in natural juice and avoid fruits canned in heavy syrup.

Poor Beverage Choices and High Blood Sugar

Regular consumption of sugar sweetened beverages, such as soda, fruit punch, sports drinks, flavored fruit drinks, high sugar tea, lattes, and coffee drinks, etc., contributes to total daily sugar/carbohydrate intake. High sugar beverages are also big contributors to excess calorie intake, unwanted weight gain and obesity, which is a risk factor for type 2 diabetes.

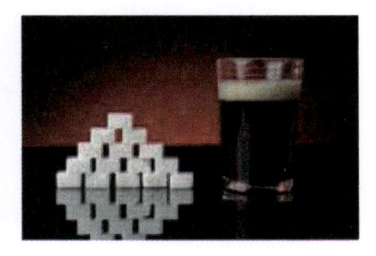

Sodas are made with high fructose corn syrup, a type of sugar made from cornstarch that has been treated with enzymes to produce a sweeter low-cost syrup.[25] High fructose corn syrup loads the body with sugar as shown in photo bellow. The small can soda contains about ten teaspoons of sugar, and the larger size bottle contains about sixteen teaspoons of sugar. Clear sodas, orange sodas, and other fruit flavored sodas contains just about the same amount of sugar as the dark sodas. Food companies use famous athletes and famous actors to advertise this high sugar beverages making them more appealing especially to teenagers and young adults. The truth is, frequently consuming beverages that contain twelve to sixteen teaspoons of sugar is an unhealthy habit and could lead to obesity and other health problems. The best and healthiest beverage choice is pure water, no additives, no sugar, no caffeine. The recommended water intake is about eight cups daily. Drink more as needed especially during intense physical activities or in hot weather days. The ancestral diet described in chapter 1 did not include any high sugar beverages.

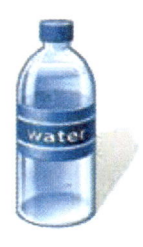

Glycemic Index of Foods

Glycemic index (GI) is a measure of how quickly different type of carbohydrate foods are broken down, digested, and turned into blood sugar. Glycemic index

---

[25] Rolfes, Pinna, and Whitney, 120.

compares foods to pure glucose which has a GI measure of 100. The higher the food GI, the quicker that food turns into blood sugar. Foods with high fiber content such as whole grains, beans, lentils and vegetables have lower glycemic index below 55 and helps maintain healthy blood sugar levels but processed foods such as white breads, white rice, and pastries made with white flour ranks in the ranges of 70 or higher on glycemic index charts and results in poor blood sugar control.

> *Low GI*: Foods that rank below 55 on the GI charts produce better gradual rise in blood sugar levels.
> *Intermediate*: Foods with GI range between 55 and 69 moderate rise in blood sugar.
> *High*: Foods with GI range of 70 or above results in blood sugar spikes, poor control of blood sugars.

Physical Activity Level and Diabetes Management

Exercise is an important aspect of diabetes management or controlling blood sugars. Physical activity includes all manner of activities and exercises from gym workouts to playing sports, taking a brisk walk in nature trails, or a very active job.

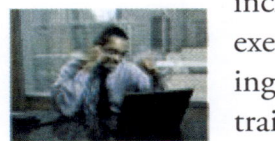

Regular physical activity has multiple health benefits. It helps reduce body fat, increases muscle mass, and helps maintain healthy body weight. Exercise improves the body's ability to utilize insulin and helps improves blood sugar control. It lowers the risk of heart disease and stroke by improving blood pressure and by lowering LDL levels/bad cholesterol in the blood.[26] The type of jobs performed contributes to daily energy and carbohydrates requirements.[27] People who work in factories moving and lifting heavy items or farm workers cultivating and tiling land, picking coffee or tea, and lifting bags of farm produce need more calories and carbohydrates than sedentary workers such as office secretaries or computer desk job workers. Daily carbohydrate needs are based on individual physical activity level, their age, weight, and gender. Recommended carbohydrate intake ranges from three to four servings (forty-five to sixty grams) for women, and four to five servings (sixty to seventy-five grams) for men.[28] See table 2B for serving sizes.

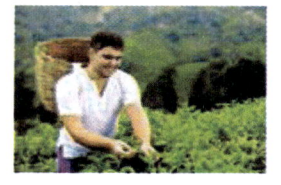

> *Highly active men and women need additional two servings of carbohydrates per meal.*

---

[26] Brown-Riggs and Jeffries, 145.
[27] https://www.niddk.nih.gov/health-information/diabetes/overview/diet-eating-physical-activity/carbohydrate-counting.
[28] https://www.cdc.gov/diabetes/managing/eat-well/diabetes-and-carbohydrates.html.

Table 2B. Carbohydrate Foods Serving Sizes
Each serving provides about fifteen grams of carbohydrates.

Starches	Fruits	Milk and Yogurt	Other
<ul><li>1 slice bread, white</li><li>½ small chapati, roti, tortilla</li><li>½ cup cooked porridge, oatmeal, cooked cereal</li><li>medium mandazi, kaimati</li><li>½ cup maize/corn, githeri, and mukimo</li><li>½ cup potatoes, sweet potatoes, yams</li><li>½ cup cooked bananas and plantains</li><li>1 cup ugali and millet ugali, 1 cup sima, 1 cup phaleche, 1cup African yams, arrow roots, cassava, and thicker cassava fufu</li><li>1 cup brown or white rice, pilau, jollof rice, and noodles=45 grams of carbs per cup*</li><li>½ cup beans and lentils, pigeon peas, green peas, chickpeas, hummus (also contains protein)</li></ul>	*Medium size*<ul><li>orange</li><li>apple</li><li>small banana</li><li>½ cup pineapple</li><li>pear, plum, peach, apricot</li><li>1 cup melons (water melon, cantaloupe, papaya, honey dew)</li><li>berries—1 cup strawberries, blueberries, raspberries, mulberries, currants</li><li>½ cup grape, black currant, cherries</li><li>raisins—2 tbsp,</li><li>½ pomegranate,</li><li>½ cup pineapple</li><li>½ mango</li></ul>	<ul><li>1 cup whole or low-fat milk</li><li>1 cup yogurt</li><li>1 cup milkshake</li><li>1 cup maziwa lala/kefir or buttermilk</li></ul>	Mixed Dishes & Casseroles made with maize with beans or lentils Soups made with beans and potatoes or noodles 1 tbsp sugar, honey or agave, jelly, and pancake syrup restrict Cakes, cupcakes, donuts, white chapatis, cookies, brownies, pastries, pies, pizza Beverages<ul><li>sodas</li><li>wines</li><li>beer</li></ul>

Non-Carbohydrate Foods

Meats/Protein	Vegetables	Fats
- *all* fish: tilapia, salmon, Nile perch, shrimp, crabs, tuna, etc. - chicken and turkey - beef - lamb and goat meat - pork - eggs - soy/tofu - cottage cheese - cheese - *Other*: nuts, peanut butter, and almond butter are high in fat	- cabbages - broccoli - kale - spinach - collards/sukuma wiki - all leafy greens: pumpkin, cassava nettles, njugu leaves, potato leaves, etc. - carrots - lettuce - cucumbers - peppers/red and green - mushrooms - onions - okra - zucchini - asparagus - garlic and other spices - other greens and vegetables not listed	*Healthy fat* Olive oil, canola oil, avocado, corn vegetable, sunflower and soybean oils *Other fats* Macadamia, cashews, peanuts, walnuts, and all other nuts - avocados mustard *Less healthy fats* - butter - mayonnaise - bacon - sour cream - half-and-half margarines

Jimmy's Blood Sugar Success Story

Take a hypothetical case of a person who we shall call Jimmy who was experiencing uncontrolled blood sugars with a very high hemoglobin A1c of 14%. The doctor referred him to a nutritionist to get help with his diet and healthy meal planning.

In his first session with the nutritionist, Jimmy explained about the changes he had made in his diet. He had stopped eating red meats and was eating only chicken and fish but had not seen any improvement in blood sugar readings. Upon reviewing Jimmy's diet history, the nutritionist found his diet to be heavy in carbohydrates, such as white rice, white bread, fried plantains, fruits, yogurt, and fufu, which is a starchy food made from cassava or yams with the consistency of mashed potatoes. Jimmy was eating too many carbohydrate servings in one meal. The nutritionist recommendations included reduced portions of fufu and plantains, changed from white rice and white bread to whole grains, brown rice, increase bean meals and non-starchy vegetables, such as green collards, spinach, broccoli, and cabbages for both lunch and dinner meals. The nutritionist also provided him a list of healthy carbohydrate foods and noncarbohydrate foods. Jimmy was surprised that his fruits, plantains, and yogurt were carbohydrate foods but was ready to make changes. The nutritionist also encouraged Jimmy to start exercising for 30 minutes 3-5 days a week. He agreed to follow both recommendations and made plans to start walking three days a week.

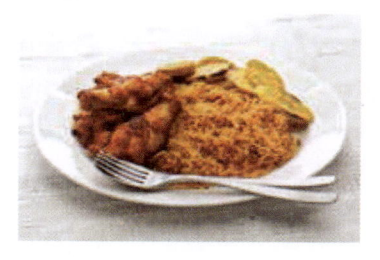

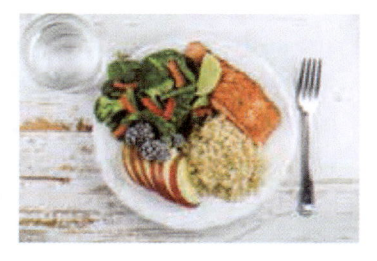

A month later, when Jimmy returned for his follow-up, he was excited about how the small changes he made in his diet and exercise had made such a big difference in his blood sugars. His fasting blood sugar reading had dropped from above 200 to a range of 105–110 every morning. He also reported being more energetic when he takes his walk and was very grateful that he was no longer frustrated with his meals and blood sugars. About three months later, when he had another blood test, his A1c results was 8%, a big drop from his last A1c of 14%. Jimmy was very excited about his improved A1c and his overall health. He left confident that he could enjoy his meals, control his blood sugar, and continue to improve his A1c to healthy levels.

Maintaining Healthy Blood Sugar Levels

Diagnosis of diabetes and recommended change in food and beverage choices, plus the home blood sugar testing or monitoring may seem a bit overwhelming to some people. However, taking medications as prescribed by your doctor and making simple changes in food choices results in quick improvements of blood sugar levels. It's highly important to discontinue drinking sweetened beverages, consuming sweet snacks as both are sources of hidden sugars. Whether the beverage is soda, caramel coffee and tea drinks, or alcoholic drink-mixes they all raise blood sugar levels. Choose drinks with no added sugar, such as sparkling water, unsweetened tea and coffee drinks, and moringa tea. Moringa leaf products are great in lowering blood sugar levels.

Restrict refined and sweetened breakfast cereals and pastries. Include vegetables such as spinach, cooked nettles, or kale in health shakes and use less fruits to reduced carbohydrates. Increase vegetables and whole grains with lunch and dinner meals. Use "The Healthy Plate" photo as guide. Make about one-third of your plate vegetables. Serving vegetables before other foods helps reduce portions of carbohydrate foods, such rice, potatoes, noodles, etc. on the plate. Restrict high fat meats and fried foods and use fish, chicken, and other white meats, bean, and lentil meals more often.

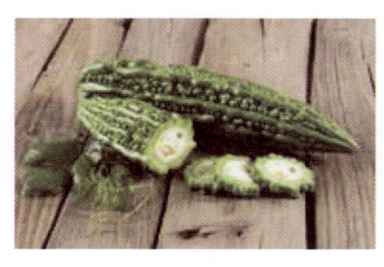

Certain vegetables and spices when used in combination with a healthy diet provides powerful effects in lowering blood sugar naturally. Cinnamon consumed regularly has many health benefits in the body including blood sugar control. Add cinnamon sticks or powder to a cup of chai tea or sprinkle cinnamon powder on buttered whole grain toast, cooked oatmeal, millet uji, and in rice pilau helps regulate blood sugar. Using garlic, ginger, and turmeric in stews or cooked vegetables also helps lower or regulate blood sugar levels. Vegetables such as kalera / bitter gourd and moringa leaves are great additions to the diet and powerful in controlling blood sugars. Kalera is served as a side dish, added to stews, or mixed with other vegetables during cooking. Remove kalera seeds before cooking and before adding small amounts of kalera cubes to health shakes. Kalera seeds are too strong and bitter especially for young children. Moringa leaves are used in many African countries as a powdered superfood added to baby foods, mashed potatoes and hot cereals and porridge due to its high protein and mineral contents. Moringa cooks like kale or collard green and makes a great side dish served with ugali, sima, or fufu.

Lon-term uncontrolled diabetes is known to cause severe damages in the body. It affects vital organs, such as kidneys leading to kidney dialysis, eye damage that could lead to blindness, nerve damage that leads to limb amputations and many other health problems. Prevention of diabetes, and reversing or improving blood sugars to healthy levels for those diagnosed with diabetes are both highly important. Taking medications as prescribed by your doctor, following a healthy balanced diet with a variety of vegetables, combined with regular physical activity results in improved healthy blood sugar levels and prevents the painful damages of uncontrolled diabetes.

CHAPTER 3

Cancer Preventive and Cancer-Fighting Nutrition

Cancer is the second leading cause of death worldwide and continues to increase at an alarming rate. Cancer has overtaken cardiovascular disease and is currently the leading cause of death in many parts of the world.[29] The most common cause of death from cancer is lung cancer, which has been attributed to tobacco smoke, followed by colorectal, stomach, liver, and breast cancers. Based on the 2016 Kenya National Guidelines for Cancer Management, cancer ranks third as the leading cause of mortality in the country after infectious diseases and cardiovascular diseases. The report recommends raising public awareness on major causes or risk factors of cancer, recommends providing Kenyans with education on ways to reduce cancer risk factors such as

---

[29] World Cancer Research Fund, 13.

cigarette smoke and harmful alcohol use, reducing exposure to air pollutants, and reducing excess body weight.[30]

Among the Kenyan communities, it's common to hear of family members spending all their savings or even selling their valued properties to cover the high cost of treatments either in private hospitals or in seeking better health care out of the country. Whether their loved ones receive cancer treatments in locally or receive treatments in other countries, many families have experienced the devastation and frustration of losing a loved one to cancer. This devastation is experienced by many families in Sub Saharan African countries. My family went through the same devastating tragedy after losing our youngest sister to cancer, which led to my increased interest in cancer prevention through nutrition and lifestyle change.

What Is Cancer?

Cancer is a collective term used to describe a disease initiated by change or disruption of normal cells causing them to start abnormal growth and multiplication. Cancerous cells could be triggered by either exposure to environmental carcinogenic agents, genetic cell damage, or poor lifestyle choices. This change causes a breakdown in cell communication channels which causes healthy functioning cells to be cut off from the normal cell chain of command. The left-out cell becomes a rogue cell in the

---

[30] National Guidelines for Cancer Management Kenya Report 2013–2016, http://www.kehpca.org/wp-content/uploads/National-Cancer-Treatment-Guidelines2.pdf.

body, and it starts to fight for its own survival. However, survival of the rogue cell depends on an environment that is favorable to its growth. If the body has a cancer promoting environment, the cancer cell starts its own mutation with abnormal growth and multiplication faster than that of normal cells.[31] To give an analogy of cancer cell growth, a rogue cell is comparable to a seed planted in the ground. The seed requires adequate water and sunlight for its germination and growth. Without water and sunlight, that seed will either remain in the ground dormant or it dries up. However, with the right environment that seed will germinate and grow into a big plant or tree. Just like a seed, the rogue precancerous cell will not grow or multiply unless the body environment allows cancer growth.[32]

It is common for rogue cells to form in a lifetime but not every rogue cell in the body turns cancerous. Research has proven that cancer cells only flourish when there are cancer promoters or cancer-friendly environment in the body to allow their growth. This simple but powerful statement indicates that making changes that create cancer-unfriendly environment in the body would cause precancerous cells to die or remain dormant. Some of the common cancer promoting or cancer friendly environments include the following:

- Exposure to chemical and environmental pollutants.

---

[31] Richard Béliveau and Denis Gingras, *Foods That Fight Cancer: What to Eat to Reduce Your Risk*, 57.
[32] Campbell and Campbell II, 42.

- Exposure to carcinogenic agents such as cigarette smoke.
- Excess weight or obesity. Fats cell overloaded with fat behave like magnets, attracting inflammatory cells from the immune system causing low chronic inflammation. Chronic body inflammation enables rogue cells to establish a new network of blood vessels to supply their nutrient needs, thereby allowing rogue cells to start abnormal cancer growth.[33]
- Heavy consumption of alcohol over long durations is associated with many health problems, and despite the few known benefits red wine, high alcohol consumption is a cause of too many diseases such as fatty liver, alcoholic liver disease, liver cirrhosis, and a cause of cancers such as liver cancer, breast cancer, and cancers of the upper digestive tract. While red wine is known to have some healthy benefits in the body, we cannot forget the list of diseases caused by high alcohol intake. It's advisable to limit intake of beers, liquor, and wine.

Cancer Preventive Environments

Creating an environment that destroys precancerous cells in the body starts with preventive measures such as avoiding toxic fumes from tobacco smoke, including secondhand smoke, avoiding exposure to toxic environments and industrial air pollution, and maintaining a

---

[33] Béliveau and Gingras, 43.

healthy weight through healthy diets and physical activity. Based on the latest research report from World Cancer Research Fund (WCRF), the types of foods we eat, how physically active we are, and carrying excess body weight are factors that influence the risk of cancer.[34] The good news is that all three factors are things that we could easily change or modify to reduce the risk of cancer.

Diets high in plant foods are not only great for maintaining a healthy body weight, but they also contain molecules that help decrease the risk of developing cancer. Over the years, we have known about the benefits of vitamins and minerals in disease prevention. However, in recent years, research in nutritional sciences has shed light on other powerful nutrients found in plant foods. Besides providing the body with vitamins and minerals, plant foods provide fiber, phytonutrients, and antioxidants, which are physiologically active compounds proven to prevent chronic diseases including cancer. Phytonutrients, also known as phytochemicals are powerful antioxidant molecules with drug-like properties that have been referred to by scientists as "chemo preventive properties" due to their ability to hinder or interfere with development of cancer cells in the body.[35]

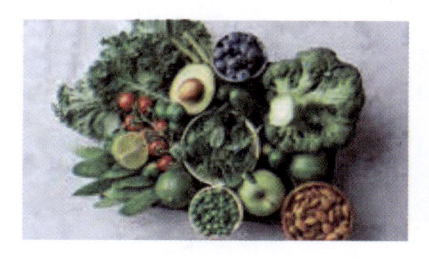

---

[34] World Cancer Research Fund.
[35] Béliveau and Gingras, 57.

> *Phyto*: Greek word for plant
> Physiologically active compounds: Compounds that impact and support normal body functions and provide disease fighting properties
> Antioxidants: Nutrients that help protect the body from unsafe molecules that are harmful to body cells.

Phytonutrients at Work

Preventive nutrition means consuming plant foods on a daily basis to maintain body environment that prevents cancer growth. It's highly important that we consume a variety of plant foods containing these powerful compounds to provide the body with weapons needed to fight cancer. Antioxidants and phytonutrients help get rid of harmful agents that cause cell damage. These molecules also create an environment in the body that is unfriendly to cancer cells, and halters growth of microscopic cancerous cells by keeping them inactive. The body is capable of destroying these frequently forming rogue cells. The capability to fight and remove the precancerous cells requires continuous consumption of plant foods, which empowers the body to keep rogue cells dormant preventing tumor growth and by destroying and removing the rogue cells through a natural process known as cell apoptosis.[36]

---

[36] Béliveau and Gingras, 33.

> *Apoptosis*: body's natural removal of damaged and abnormal cancerous cells without causing damage to the normal body cells.
> *Phytochemicals*: naturally occurring plant molecules that provide the various colors, tastes, and aromas in plant foods. Phytochemicals are referred to as chemo-preventive molecules due to their cancer fighting benefits.

Nutrients in the Cabbage Group of Vegetables

Research on cancer-fighting molecules in plant foods rates cabbage and the cabbage family of vegetables as some of the most potent cancer-fighting foods. The cabbage group includes the commonly used green cabbage, the curly and crinkly green cabbages, the purple cabbages, and brussels sprouts. These vegetables contain phytochemicals that help reduce cancer-related hormones that trigger cancer cell and tumor growth.[37] Other phytonutrients in cabbages include minerals that helps heal stomach and duodenal ulcers. Cabbages contain molecules that help stimulate production of the antioxidant glutathione in the body. Glutathione helps boost the body's immune system and plays a role in liver detoxification.

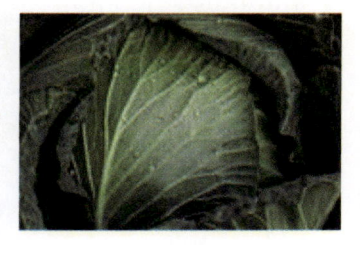

---

[37] Béliveau and Gingras, 83.

Other vegetables in the cabbage family with similar cancer-fighting molecules includes broccoli, cauliflower, kale, and collard greens. These vegetables contain large quantities of powerful anticancer compounds. Cabbages, kale, cauliflower, broccoli, and collards are commonly served as side dishes. Kale and collard greens are commonly served with ugali in East African countries and also served with South African pap, or either cassava sima, yams, fufu, and other dishes in many cultures. Cauliflower is used as a tasty side dish, and because of its soft consistency, cauliflower is easily mixed in foods such as mashed potatoes to reduce carbohydrate content and to increase nutrients. Purple cabbages, kale, and broccoli are also used as ingredients in vegetable salads for added color, flavor, and to boost phytonutrients

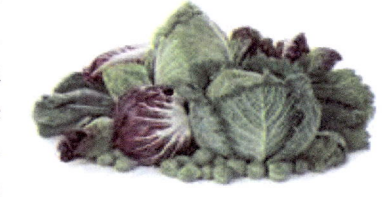

> Phytonutrients and antioxidants provides the following health benefits*[38]
>
> - They stimulate the immune system to fight against diseases
> - They help block harmful substances and pollutants that we may breathe in from becoming carcinogens
> - Reduces body inflammation known to allow cancer growth, thereby blocking cancer cell growth
> - Reduces damage to cells that could lead to rogue cells and growth into cancerous cells
> - They help trigger death of damaged cells through apoptosis before they could multiply or grow to tumors
> - They help regulate hormones in the body and reduce cancer-related hormones
> - They help prevent DNA damage and help with DNA repair

Red, Yellow and Orange Color Vegetables

Two major phytonutrients in these group of foods include lycopene and beta-carotene powerful cancer fighting molecules. Both phytonutrients provide the body with antioxidants, anti-inflammatory effects, high amounts of vitamin A and C, nutrients that help hinder growth of cancer cells, and reduces the risk of many types

---

[38] Kate Ramos, *Healing Foods: Eat Your Way to a Healthier Life*, 52.

of cancers including lung, prostate, and breast cancers.[39] Lycopene is found mostly in food with red pigments, such as tomatoes, radishes, red bell peppers, rhubarb, watermelon, red berries guavas, etc. Beta-carotene is found in large amounts in food with orange-yellow pigments, such as orange sweet potatoes, pumpkins papayas, peaches, mangoes, oranges. Vegetables high in these phytonutrients are commonly used as ingredients in soups and casseroles. They could also be added to other foods to boost nutrient intake. Adding pumpkins to chapati dough add a boost of vitamins A, vitamin C, and lycopene while adding a hint of beautiful orange color to chapatis. Use a combination of red and orange color vegetables to make a dish of roasted vegetables. (See sample recipe below.) Add pomegranate fruit to your vegetables and fruit smoothies to boost cancer-fighting antioxidants with your breakfast. Pomegranate seeds also contain antiviral properties. Make a spinach pineapple and papaya smoothie, add about ten papaya seeds in the shake to boost vitamins, minerals, and antioxidant properties. Papaya seeds are mostly used in spices and add peppery taste to foods.

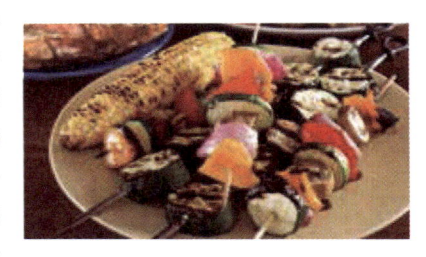

---

[39] DK Publishers, p. 65.

Recipe: *Starchy Tubers and Vegetables Mix*

Ingredients
1 c. sliced carrots
1 c. diced pumpkin or butternut squash
1 medium white or purple sweet potato, cut in chunks
1 large green pepper, sliced lengthwise
1 c. grape tomatoes
1 large purple onion, cut lengthwise
1 garlic bulb cut lengthwise
(Change to your favorite vegetables as needed)
2 tbs. olive oil or vegetable oil,
Pinch of salt
Pinch of black pepper
Dry spices such as basil and thyme and rosemary

Place all vegetables in large bowl. Add olive oil and salt. Toss to coat vegetables with oil. Place in large baking dish. Sprinkle with spices and bake at 425 degree for about 45 minutes till the starchy vegetables are soft

Purple and Blue Fruits and Vegetables

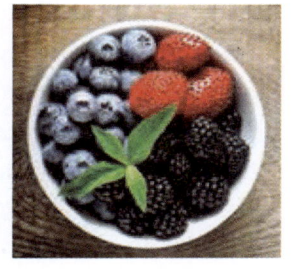

The purple and blue color groups of vegetables and fruits, including purple cabbages, purple grapes, plums, blueberries, and blackberries, etc., are high in flavonoids such as anthocyanin the antioxidant that gives fruits that deep blue-purple color seen in blueberries and blackberries. Blueberries and other similar color berries contain phytochemicals and antioxidants proven to stop growth of cancer cells.[40] Adding berries to oatmeal, yogurt, or fruit and vegetables salads is a great way to add daily intake of phytonutrients. Recommended daily intake of vegetables is about 2 cups cooked vegetables for adults. Vegetables are very low in calories, and consuming more than the minimum recommendation not only helps prevent unwanted weight but also boosts intake of vitamins, minerals, fiber, and phytonutrients in the diet.

Phytonutrients in Green and Black Tea

Tea is commonly served as a hot or cold beverage in many countries. Hot tea is served in almost every home and restaurant in Eastern Africa and in many other African countries. Spices such as ginger, cinnamon and cardamom are added to chai as desired. Chai tea could be sweetened with honey or sugar as desired. Chai tea is popular in many African countries, Middle East, India, Britain, Caribbean islands. Tea is also consumed in many countries as iced tea or green tea. Green and black teas are both products of same tea leaves; however, the processing time of black tea is longer than that of green tea. Black tea is allowed to be more oxidized turning tea leaves into a bronze black color and results in darker tea leaves. Green tea takes a shorter time to process and yields light green tea leaves and retains more phytonutrients than black tea. Studies have shown that green tea

---

[40] DK Publishers, 30.

contains high levels of antioxidants and phytochemicals with anticancer properties proven to prevent development of breast, prostate, skin, lung, stomach, and colon cancers.[41] Green tea is simply made by steeping tea leaves or teabags in a kettle or a cup of hot water for about 2 minutes, and adding either ginger, lemon and honey as desired. To obtain optimal benefits from green tea, drink two to three cups hot or cold tea daily. In recent years Kenyan tea farmers started locally owned tea factories which increased farmer's incomes from tea sales. Some of the farmers also use farm fresh tea leaves to make home processed tea. Home processed tea yields tea leaves that are in between black and green tea leaves and makes a tasty cup of chai tea.

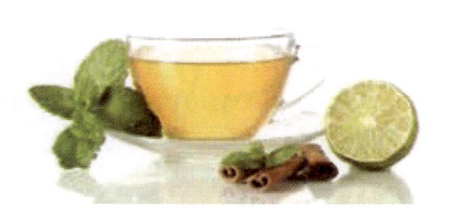

Food research shows that scientists have identified thousands of healing nutrients, and antioxidants in various plant foods, and indicated the importance of regular consumption of Plant foods to equip the body with these powerful phytochemicals as shown in Table 5. The chart lists some of the phytochemicals, identifies food sources and potential health benefits.

---

[41] Béliveau and Gingras, 137–138.

Red Meats and Processed Foods

The latest report from American Cancer Institute and World Cancer Research Fund recommends moderate consumption of red meats. The report recommends that intake of red meats be limited to 300-500 grams or 12-18 ounces per week. This might seem to be a big change among many Africans who are used to eating fire-grilled red meats commonly referred to as "nyama choma" in East Africa, it may also be a big change for people who enjoy western-type diets where restaurants serve 9 oz (ounce) steaks per plate. The report also indicates that consuming more than 18 ounces of red meats in a week has been shown to increase the risk of colon and rectal cancers. Research evidence shows that high consumption of animal proteins increases the risk of colon, breast, and prostate cancers. However, plant foods not only provide the body with adequate amounts of protein and iron but also provide the added benefits of cancer-fighting phytonutrients. Consuming protein from foods such as beans, lentils, chickpeas, soybeans, nuts etc. helps fight cancer and tumor development in body cells.[42]

---

[42] T. Colin Campbell and Thomas Campbell II, *The China Study: Startling Implications for Diet, Weight Loss and Long-Term Health*, 57.

Table 3. Phytochemical Chart—Health Benefits of Phytonutrients[43]

Phytochemical(s)	Plant Source	Health Benefits
Carotenoids—reds and orange colors (such as beta-carotene, lycopene, lutein, zeaxanthin)	Red, orange, and green fruits and vegetables including carrots, cooked tomatoes, sweet potatoes, pumpkins, apricots, cantaloupe, peach, mangos, oranges papayas, watermelons, broccoli, and leafy greens	Inhibits cancer cell growth, works as antioxidants and improves immune response
Flavonoids (such as anthocyanins and quercetin)	Apples, citrus fruits, onions, soybeans, soy products (such as tofu, soy milk, edamame, etc.), coffee, green tea, and regular black tea	Inhibits inflammation and tumor growth; aids immunity and boosts production of detoxifying enzymes in the body

---

[43] Jean LaMantia and Neil Berinstein, *Cancer Treatment Nutrition Guide and Cookbook*, 120.

Indoles and glycosylates (sulforaphane)	Cruciferous vegetables (broccoli, cabbage, collard greens, kale, cauliflower, and brussels sprouts)	Induces detoxification of carcinogens, limits production of cancer-related hormones, blocks carcinogens and prevents tumor growth
Isoflavones (daidzein and genistein)	Soybeans and soy products (tofu, soy milk, edamame)	Inhibits tumor growth, limited production of cancer-related hormones, and generally works as an antioxidant
Isothiocyanates	Cruciferous vegetables (broccoli, cabbage, collard greens, kale, cauliflower, and brussels sprouts)	Induces detoxification of carcinogens, blocks tumor growth, and works as an antioxidant

Polyphenols (such as ellagic acid and resveratrol)	Green tea, grapes, wine, berries, citrus fruits, apples, whole grains, and peanuts	Prevents cancer formation, prevents inflammation, and works as an antioxidant
Terpenes such as limonene and carnosol	Cherries, citrus fruit peel, seasoning rosemary	Protects cells from becoming cancerous, slows cancer cell growth, strengthens immune function, limits production of cancer-related hormones, fights viruses, works as an antioxidant

One Day Sample Menu

Healthy meals should include whole grains, vegetables, and fruits high in phytonutrients and, whenever possible, cooked with spices that provided anticancer effects.

Breakfast Meal: Egg and Vegetable Omelet
Vegetable omelet made with two eggs, one cup baby spinach, ¼ of a small chopped purple onion, ½ cup chopped green and red peppers, pinch of salt, black pepper, pinch of turmeric. Served with one cup hot green tea, two slices whole grain toast with peanut butter, one cup blackberries

Cancer-fighting foods in this breakfast meal include the three different color vegetables—green and red peppers, tomatoes. Seasonings: a combination of black pepper and turmeric is a powerful cancer fighter and is also good for reducing body inflammation. Blackberries and green tea are high in antioxidants and cancer-fighting molecules.

Lunch Meal: Quick Maize, Red Beans Vegetable and Avocado Salad
Ingredients: 1 cup baby spinach (washed), 1.5 cups cooked red bean and maize mix, 1/2 cup sliced cucumbers, 1.2 medium-sized avocado, 1/2 cup cherry tomatoes, 1/4 cup purple onion (thinly sliced), 2 tablespoons grated cheese, pinch of salt, and pinch of black pepper.

Preparation: Line large-size plate with baby spinach, add bean and maize mix on top of spinach, add cherry tomatoes and cucumbers to top maize and beans/githeri mix, cut avocado into small slices, place avocado on top of the salad mix, and sprinkle with grated cheese. Add salt and pepper as desired.

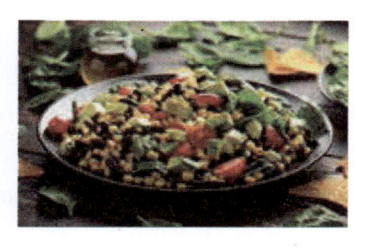

Desert: one large mango cut into cubes, water.

Cancer-fighting foods: *red kidney beans and all vegetables*

Dinner Meal: Lentil and Vegetable Soup with Chapati

One bowl lentil vegetable soup (see recipe below) served with a whole grain chapati.

Desert: fresh pear, tall glass of water

Cancer fighters: *all ingredients in the soup. Turmeric is a powerful spice in cancer cell destruction through apoptosis.*

Snack: one cup mixed berry, one cup yogurt.

Cancer fighters: *Berries contain large amounts of vitamin C and powerful cancer fighting phytonutrients. Include blackberries, red berries and blue berries as available. Serve berries as a snack, added to breakfast cereals and fruit salads.*

Lentil soup

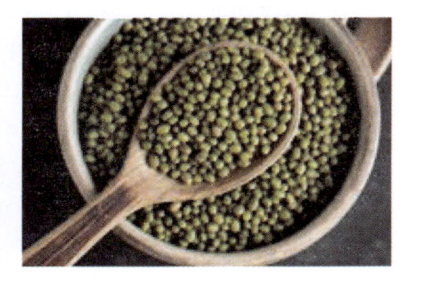

Ingredients: One cup green mung beans(ndengu) rinsed, ½ medium purple onion diced, 4 gloves garlic chopped, 1 tsp grated ginger, 1small stalk celery diced, 1 cup diced carrots, 1 medium 1 cup diced red peppers, 2 tablespoons chopped cilantro, ¼ tsp turmeric, ¼ tsp salt, 1/8 tsp black pepper, 2 tablespoons olive oil or vegetable oil, 5 cups water or (chicken broth optional)

Instructions: In a medium saucepan, add oil, onions, ginger and garlic and Sautee on low heat until onions are soft, add turmeric, salt and black pepper and stir seasonings, add celery and carrots, stir and cook for 2 minutes, add red peppers and cilantro, stir vegetables and cook on low heat for another 2 minutes. Add lentils and water and cook on high heat to bring lentils to a boil for about 2 minutes, reduce to low heat and cook covered for about 30-40 minutes or until lentils are soft. Serve with whole grain chapati. Chapati could be substituted with brown rice. Add spices or hots as needed.

Cancer fighter includes: *All vegetables, mung beans, garlic, ginger and turmeric*

Mango Papaya Avocado Berry Salad

3 cups papaya, 2 cups diced mango, and 1 medium avocado diced into cubes. 2 cups black berries. Place diced papaya, mango and avocado in a large dish, toss lightly. Top with blackberries. Makes a great tasting and refreshing afternoon pick-me-up snack, loaded with healthy fats, vitamin E, and the antioxidant glutathione from the avocado. Mango and papaya are both high in vitamin A, B, and C. Papayas and mangos are also high in phytochemicals lycopene and beta-carotenes, which work as anti-

oxidants in the body. Mangos contain plant hormones shown to have protective effects against prostate cancer.[44]

Chicken Vegetable Stir-Fry

Ingredients: 1 pound or ½ kg cut up chicken breast, 1 cup sliced carrots, 1 cup diced green peppers, 2 cups broccoli florets, 1 medium tomato, 2 tablespoons olive oil, ¼ cup diced onion, 1/2 tsp grated ginger, 1 tablespoon diced garlic, pinch of salt, pinch of black pepper, 1 table spoon low sodium soy sauce.

Instructions: In medium pot, add oil, onions, garlic, salt, black pepper, and ginger. Stir-fry till slightly withered. Add chicken and stir-fry for five to ten minutes. (Farm raised or free range chicken will need more cooking time of about 20-25 minutes.) Add carrots and stir and cook for two to three minutes. Add green peppers and tomatoes. Continue to stir-fry for another three minutes. Add small amounts of water only as needed. Add broccoli last. Add soy sauce and cook for another 2-3 minutes. Chicken stir-fry tastes great served over steamed rice.

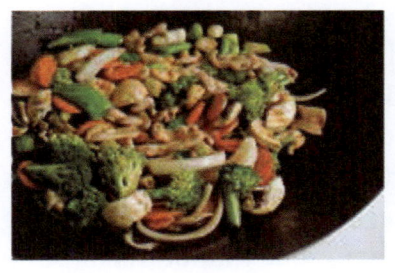

---

[44] Ramos, 43.

Adding Phytonutrients During Cancer Treatments

During active chemotherapy and radiation treatments, the body's immune system could become weakened, leading to reduced ability to fight against bacteria and viruses. Recommendations for people on active cancer treatments is to avoid eating open deli meats, avoid salads, and eat cooked vegetables, eat peeled or canned fruit to help reduce any chance of food-borne illnesses. Some people may also experience nausea and poor appetite during cancer treatments. Consume foods that are easy to chew and easy to digest, such as baked foods, soft cooked casseroles, and soups to help reduce nausea, improve intake of essential nutrient and phytonutrients in meals.

During active cancer treatments, regular consumption of foods high in phytochemicals adds continuous bombardment against cancerous cells and tumors. The plant foods listed below contain hefty amounts of powerful cancer fighting phytonutrients.

- Raw nuts, especially macadamia and almonds.
- Millet, sorghum, flax seeds or flax flour.
- Moringa leaves, moringa leaf powder, and moringa seeds.
- Cruciferous vegetables
- Proteins from beans—red beans, lima beans, mung beans, and fava beans or broad beans.

There's strong evidence that a healthy diet high in plant foods is cancer protective. World Cancer Research

Fund (WCRF) recommend a diet high in plant proteins and high in fiber from whole grains foods, beans legumes, fruits, and vegetables. The recommendations also include diets low in animal proteins and especially low in red meats, a diet low in sugar from foods, snacks, or sugar sweetened beverages, such as soda. Consuming plant-based diet provides the body with adequate proteins, healthy fats, vitamins, high amounts of anti-inflammatory phytonutrients and antioxidants known to help fight various cancers.[45]

The fight against cancer requires both avoiding foods and beverages that promote cancer-friendly body environment and continuously feeding the body with plant foods high in antioxidants and phytonutrients that help detoxify the body, prevent cancer cell growth, destroy and remove cancerous cells, while promoting growth of new healthy cells and providing healing and restoration in the body.

---

[45] World Cancer Research Fund, American Institute of Cancer Research. "Diet Nutrition, Physical Activity and Cancer: A Global Perspective," 2018, 54.

CHAPTER 4

Heart Health

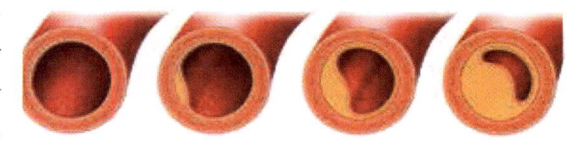

The terms heart disease and cardiovascular disease are used to describe various health problems that affects the heart. Heart disease includes illnesses that affects the vessels that surround the heart called coronary arteries, which supply oxygen and nutrients to the heart muscles. It also includes conditions that affect the network of blood vessels that carry blood in and out of the heart, delivering oxygen and nutrients to the entire body. The most common type of heart disease is coronary heart disease which affects the vessels that feed the heart. This health problem is mainly caused by fatty cholesterol deposits and accumulation on the inner walls of coronary arteries and other blood vessels. Cholesterol build up is a gradual process which forms plaque-like build-up gets wedged in on the walls of coronary arteries. High cholesterol in the blood is a major cause of plaque buildup in the arterial walls, resulting in narrowing of blood vessels and causing reduced flow of oxygen-rich blood to the heart muscle which could lead to heart attack.[46] Other causes of plaque build-up in blood vessels includes smoking, high blood pressure, poor diets and chronic body inflammation.

Cholesterol

Cholesterol is a soft waxlike substance manufactured in the body by the liver. Cholesterol has an important role in the body as a component of all healthy cell membranes. It's needed in the body for synthesis of hormones such as aldosterone, cortisol, estrogen, and testosterone. Cholesterol is also needed for the synthesis of vitamin D, which plays a role in maintaining healthy bones and teeth and it's used for the synthesis and production of bile juice, an essential digestive juice vital for breakdown and absorption of fats.[47]

> *Cholesterol: A white waxlike substance found only in animal foods and animal-based food products.*
> *Atherosclerosis: A disease caused by fatty plaque-like cholesterol buildup inside the walls of blood vessels, leading to blockage of blood flow, depriving supply of oxygen and nutrients to cells and organs.*

---

[46] Rolfes, Pinna, and Whitney, 819.
[47] Bond Brill, 11.

Cholesterol in the blood comes from two sources: cholesterol synthesized by the liver and cholesterol from the food we consume. The liver is capable of synthesizing all the cholesterol needed in the body. When we eat high cholesterol foods, the liver makes additional cholesterol. Research in food and blood cholesterol shows that consuming diets high in animal fats and saturated fats contributes to high blood cholesterol levels, especially the LDL/bad cholesterol which is linked to heart disease.[48]

Good and Bad Cholesterol

The two major types of cholesterol in the blood are HDL and LDL referred to as the good and bad cholesterols. The difference between the two types of cholesterols is that HDL has protective effects in the body but LDL in known to produce harmful effects. For cholesterol to move through the blood, which is a liquid, the body makes protein helpers or couriers called lipoproteins that attach to cholesterol and help transport it in the blood stream. The two main lipoproteins in the body are low-density lipoproteins or LDL, and high-density lipoproteins or HDL. High density lipoprotein plays the important role of transporting cholesterol out of the arteries and moving it into the liver where it's used for body cells as needed. By moving cholesterol out of the arteries, HDL reduces plaque-like buildup in the arter-

---

[48] Campbell and Campbell II, *China Study. Revised and Expanded Edition*, 69.

ies, reducing the risk of coronary artery disease.[49] Low-density lipoproteins or LDL are the couriers of majority of cholesterol in the blood and are considered unhealthy or bad cholesterol because high levels of LDL in the blood has been linked to fatty deposits in the arteries that cause plaque-like build up in the arterial walls, referred to as atherosclerosis. Severe buildup of plaques like fatty deposits could lead to clogged arteries. This is why LDL in called bad cholesterol.

> *Lipo: Fat or lipid.*
> *Lipoproteins: Fats enveloped in proteins that allows fat/cholesterol transport in the bloodstream.*

Blood Cholesterol Tests

High blood cholesterol has no symptoms. The only way to find out what your blood cholesterol levels are is through a blood test. Medical providers usually order a blood test commonly referred to as blood lipid panel, which is completed after overnight fast. This test ana-

---

[49] Rolfes, Pinna, Whitney, 821.

lyzes blood levels of total cholesterol, LDL cholesterol, HDL cholesterol, and triglyceride levels as noted below:

Table 4A Healthy Blood Cholesterol Levels (by Age and Gender)

Demographic	Total Cholesterol	LDL	HDL
Youth age 19 years or younger	Less than 170 mg/dl	Less than 100 mg/dl	45 mg/dl or higher
Men 20 years or older	125–200mg/dl	Less than 100mg/dl	40 mg/dl or higher
Women 20 years or older	125–200 mg/dl	Less than 100 mg/dl	50 mg or higher

Source: American Heart Association[50]

Triglycerides

Triglycerides are the main types of fats in foods especially in animal food products. When we consume meals or diets containing too much fat and too many calories, the excess is stored in body fat cells as triglycerides. High triglycerides levels in the blood could lead to clogged up arteries and increase the risk of heart disease. High levels of triglycerides in the blood is also associated with inflamed pancreas or pancreatitis.[51] Triglyceride lab

---

[50] https://www.nhlbi.nih.gov/health-topics/high-blood-cholesterol
[51] Rolfes, Pinna, Whitney, 746.

results, which is completed after an overnight fast, are categorized as follows: Normal levels Less than 150 mg/dl Borderline level 150–199 mg/dl High levels 200-499 mg/dl or higher.[52] Major causes of high triglycerides levels in the blood includes high intake of processed meats, high-fat foods, high-alcohol intake and simple carbohydrates foods, such as white bread, white rice, pasta, cookies, cakes, etc. A diet low in fat and high in fiber helps lower levels of triglycerides and other blood lipids.

Cooking Oils & Cooking Fats

Choosing healthy cooking oils is an important part of heart healthy diet. Cooking oils that are liquid at room temperature are better options than solid fats in preventing heart disease. These cooking oils are generally cholesterol-free and trans-fat free. Good choices include olive oil, canola, safflower oil, avocado oil, sunflower, and other liquid oils. These cooking oils provide great health benefits when used in low heat/temperature cooking or when used as salad dressings. Coconut oil which is also cholesterol free, is a better oil for heat/high temperature cooking and provides great health benefits. Animal fats such as butter and ghee could be used sparingly in a healthy diet high in vegetables and whole grains. Include cholesterol free alternatives such as, fresh ripe avocados, peanut butter almond butter and other nut and seed butters as part of diet. Cooking lard which is sold in some African local butcheries as a low-cost cooking fat, is a high cholesterol

---

[52] Barnard, 136.

fat and should be used very sparingly or replaced with coconut oil or vegetables oils.

Trans Fats & Heart Health

Trans fats are vegetable cooking fats and breakfast spreads or margarines made from oils that are liquid at room temperature. These oils are processed to make softer, smooth consistency fats or spreads. This process of making solid fats from liquid oils, known as hydrogenation, results in soft solid fats referred to as trans fats. These types of fats have a longer shelf life than other fats.[53] Research has shown that consuming trans fats contributes to heart disease by increasing the bad cholesterol (LDL) in the body.[54] Many food companies use trans fats in snack foods such as cookies, potato chips, cakes, donuts, frozen french fries etc. due to their longer shelf life compared to other fats. Its import that we read nutrition facts on food labels to identify and restrict foods and snacks high in trans fats. Restrict processed foods and frozen foods, ready to eat frozen meals and other prepackaged foods and snacks made with trans fats.

Lowering Blood Cholesterol Naturally

Two important lifestyle changes that are used to lower blood cholesterol are low fat diets and regular physical activity, both referred to as therapeutic lifestyle change/

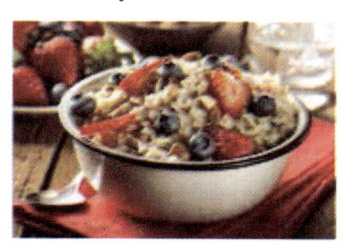

---

[53] Rolfes, Pinna, and Whitney, 146.
[54] Bond Brill, 138.

TLC. These changes are recommended by National Heart Lung and Blood Institute, American Heart Association, and many other health organizations as an important step in lowering LDL cholesterol, blood pressure, and obesity in lowering blood cholesterol levels.[55] Heart healthy therapeutic lifestyle includes regular physical activity at a moderate pace for about 30 minutes a day, 3–5 days a week, plus a healthy eating plan that reduces cholesterol, saturated fats, and helps prevent overweight and obesity. Cholesterol is found only in animal foods such as high fat meats, eggs, and whole milk and products made from whole milk such as butter, ghee, and cheese. Plants foods do not contain any cholesterol and provides the body with adequate amounts of protein and iron. Plant foods are also good sources of soluble fiber and insoluble fibers. Insoluble fiber promotes regular gut motility, prevents constipation, and bowel diseases. Soluble fiber has been proven to lower blood cholesterol.[56] Soluble fiber lowers LDL blood cholesterol by decreasing cholesterol absorption and by increasing excretion of cholesterol and bile acids out of the gut.[57] Powerful cholesterol lowering soluble fiber is found in foods such as oatmeal, millet, barley. Other foods high in soluble fiber includes beans and legumes, nuts, and vegetables such as okra, peas, and brussels sprouts.

---

[55] "Your Guide to Lowering Cholesterol," https://www.nhlbi.nih.gov/health-topics/all-publications-and-resources/your-guide-lowering-cholesterol-therapeutic-lifestyle. C
[56] Bond Brill, 48.
[57] Bond Brill, 48.

Meals and Cholesterol Content

Common meals consumed by most people in major cities and urban areas in Sub-Saharan Africa, includes high cholesterol foods. Breakfast meals may include one or more of the following items. Bread with butter, mandazi or chapati made with high cholesterol fats, eggs sausage bacon or coffee cakes and pastries made with butter. Lunch and dinner meals may also include high fat meats such as hamburgers, high fat steaks, pork ribs, or fire grilled red meats common in many African countries, referred to as "choma" in East Africa. Other high cholesterol foods include organ meats such as liver, hearts and gizzards; shrimp, crabs, lobsters and other shellfish. Frequently consuming these high cholesterol foods increases blood cholesterol levels. Replace high cholesterol meats with fish and a variety of beans meals, combined with high fiber vegetables such as egg plants, broccoli, green collards, brussels sprouts, okra, etc. Increase intake of bran from whole grains such as millet, sorghum, oats, barley and maize etc.

Regular consumption of beans, legumes, whole grains, and vegetables as part of diet provides the body with these important soluble fibers that lowers blood cholesterol naturally. Beans and lentils are also good sources of amino acids and molecules that help dilate blood vessels.

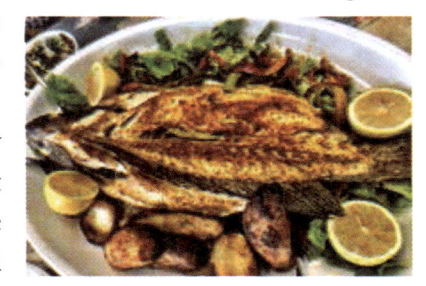

Beans make tasty nutritious meals that could be enjoyed by the whole family. Try baked beans and maize mix as breakfast meals. Make a variety of bean soups for the family. Consume more variety of bean and lentil meals for lunch and dinner. Adding beans, peas, or njahi beans to vegetable salads is a quick way to increase protein, carbohydrates, and soluble fiber, plus important vitamins and minerals. Other heart-healthy foods include omega-3 fats found in fish, such as albacore tuna, salmon, trout, king mackerel, sardines, Lake Victoria's omena, etc. and other fish, such as Nile perch, yellow-fin tuna, commonly used in South Africa, tilapia, and many other fish varieties. Using heart healthy omega-3 fats from fish, nuts, and seeds helps lower triglyceride levels in the blood, reduces inflammation in the body and in blood vessels, and improves heart health.

> *Beans*: are complete foods high in protein, carbohydrates, B vitamins, magnesium, zinc, potassium, phytonutrients and soluble fiber that helps lower blood cholesterol.

Healthy Blood Pressure and Heart Health

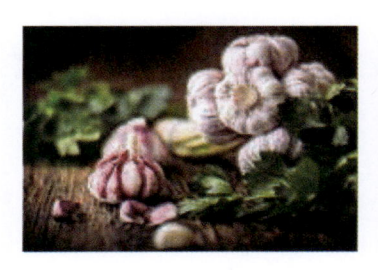

High blood pressure of hypertension is a major risk factor for heart disease. High blood pressure is also referred to as the "silent killer" due to its quiet damage to vessels and body organs without any symptoms. Blood pressure measures the force exerted against the walls of blood vessels as oxygen-rich blood is delivered from the heart to the entire body. Blood pressure is measured in two numbers, referred to as systolic and diastolic pressures. When the heart contracts and pushes blood out in the vessels, this measurement is called systolic pressure, when the heart muscle is relaxed between beats, this measurement is the diastolic pressure. Normal blood pressure measurements are 120/80 systolic over diastolic numbers. High blood pressure or hypertension is an elevated force of blood moving from the heart to blood vessels measuring above 140/90.[58]

Factors that contribute to high blood pressure in the body include obesity, lack of regular exercise, smoking, consistent stress and narrowed blood vessels from cholesterol buildup in the vessels, leading to restricted blood flow. Other contributors to high blood pressure include increased blood volume which is caused by fluid buildup in the body. Excess fluid in the body results in the heart working harder to pump blood into the vessels. High blood pressure is a major risk factor for stroke, cardiovascular disease, damage to the tiny blood vessels in kidneys, and is the second leading cause of kidney failure.[59]

---

[58] Rolfes, Pinna, and Whitney, 833.
[59] https://www.niddk.nih.gov/health-information/kidney-disease/high-blood-pressure. High Blood Pressure & Kidney Disease.

Foods That Improve Blood Pressure

Diet plays a big role in blood pressure control. Fresh fruits and vegetables help lower blood pressure while canned and processed foods such as pickles, bacon, and sausage links contributes to blood pressure to raise due to their high salt/sodium contents. There are many research studies showing importance of diet in blood pressure control, with the strongest evidence coming from DASH diet or Dietary Approaches to Stop Hypertension. This study showed that blood pressure was lowered through a diet moderate in salt intake, low cholesterol foods, low fat dairy foods, and high in whole grains, vegetables, and fruits.[60] Other strategies that help improve blood pressure include moderate weight loss for those who are overweight, reduced intake of salt, moderation in alcohol consumption, and a healthy diet containing foods that are high in the minerals potassium, magnesium, and calcium.[61] These minerals known to help lower blood pressure are readily available in foods such as beans, broccoli, kale, spinach, potatoes, pumpkins, nut, oranges, bananas, and many other vegetables and fruits.

---

[60] US Department of Health and Human Services, National Institute of Health, National Heart, Lung and Blood Institutes, *Your Guide to Lowering Your Blood Pressure with DASH*, 6–8, https://www.nhlbi.nih.gov/files/docs/public/heart/new_dash.pdf.

[61] Marla Heller, *The DASH Diet Action Plan: Proven to Lower Blood Pressure and Cholesterol without Medication*, 16, 135.

Maintaining normal blood pressure is an important measure toward improved heart health. It's important to consume more fresh foods and less processed foods due to their high contents of fat and sodium. Restrict high sodium foods such as pizza, sausages, hot dogs, soy sauce and foods made with soy sauce, noodle packets and cups of noodles. Reduce salt in cooking, and use different spices, garlic, ginger, turmeric, curry powder etc., to season meals. Recommended salt/sodium intake for adults is about 2000 mg a day and 1500 mg for people with hypertension. Consume a healthy balanced diet high in whole grains, fruits and vegetables, beans, low fat foods and moderate in salt intake for healthy blood pressure and heathy heart. Whole grains and vegetables are high in soluble fiber. They provide important B vitamins, vitamin C, E, and minerals that promote both healthy blood pressure and healthy heart. These nutrients play an important role in prevention and treatment of heart disease and are highly important for those diagnosed with high cholesterol, atherosclerosis, and those recovering from heart attack. A diet high in fiber from whole grains, vegetables, legumes, and fruits promote healthy blood-pressure levels, helps increase HDL levels in the blood while decreasing LDL cholesterol, help maintain healthy blood-sugar levels, leading to improved heart health. Keep in mind, our ancestral diets were low-fat, low-sodium, high-fiber plant-based diets.

CHAPTER 5

Losing Weight and Keeping It Off

Overweight and obesity are defined as having body weight that is higher than what is considered a healthy weight for an individual's height. Being too heavy or carrying extra body fat is often a result of either overconsumption of food, sedentary lifestyles, and for very few, people's genetics. Obesity is a known cause of chronic illnesses, such as type 2 diabetes, heart disease, hypertension, and some types of cancers. Obesity also contributes to respiratory health problems, such as sleep apnea and causes degeneration of joint cartilages and joint problems. Losing weight and maintaining a healthy weight is an important factor in prevention of chronic illnesses and for overall health and well-being.

Common New Year's resolutions in many countries comprise of weight loss, healthy eating, and resolutions to increase exercise for improved health. Many people start off the new year by implementing changes to improve their diets; they may join a gym with intentions of exercising more often to help attain their new year's weight-loss resolutions. However, these resolutions don't last long, and most people usually drop out of their diet and exercise programs and go back to their usual lifestyles within the first four to six weeks of the new year. Most people do not have a good plan in place, and with challenging schedules, they drop out of newly-implemented routines and go back to their former lifestyles and food choices, which leads to more weight gain. It's also common for people interested in weight loss to try the many available diet programs, such as high-protein, low-carbohydrates diets, keto diets, meal-replacement shakes, prepackaged home-delivered meals, etc., but no matter which diet programs they try to follow, they get tired or frustrated with the regimens or bland meals and tend to make statements like "I look forward to completing this diet program and go back to my normal meal routine." In my experience as a nutritionist, it's common for my clients to tell me their weight-loss stories of how they had lost fifteen or twenty pounds and were happy and celebrated their hard work, but a few months after they stopped dieting, they regained all the weight and ended up heavier than before the weight loss. This cycle of losing and regaining weight can be a source of frustration to many people. However, there is a way to eat healthy and lose weight without feeling frustrated.

Losing Weight and Keeping It Off

Behavior change or behavior modification plays a key role in attaining weight loss and maintaining healthy weight. Successful weight loss requires changing food choices, increasing physical activity, forming new habits that promote a balance in calories consumed and physical activity level. The following lifestyle changes results in successful weight loss:

- Healthy food shopping and food prepping
- Making healthy selections when eating out in restaurant or cafes
- Healthy beverage choices
- Mindful eating and portion control
- Regular exercise/physical activity

Healthy Food Shopping

Healthy meals for weight loss starts with the foods we bring home from the supermarket. The foods and snack items we buy becomes our diet. Making a supermarket food list of all items needed before going food shopping prevents buying on impulse and prevents bringing home foods that promote weight gain, such as cookies, cakes, sodas, and other high calorie foods that you had planned to avoid. Using a food shopping list also allows one to bring home groceries needed in the following week. Grocery shopping while hungry makes unhealthy foods and snacks appear more appetizing and appealing than when one is not hungry, it leads to buying high calorie food items that are not on your food list. Table 5A contains a list of healthy food choices and some examples of high fat high sugar foods that should be restricted due to their high calorie contents.

Table 5A.

Healthy Food Choices	Foods to Restrict or Avoid
- When shopping breakfast food include whole grains, breads, English muffins, whole grain cereal, such as cheerios, oatmeal, millet/porridge uji. - Low-fat milks, yogurts, peanut butter or almond butter. Eggs and turkey sausages - Low-fat milk, yogurts and kefir (maziwa lala). Almond and soy milk. - Buy variety of leafy vegetables and other vegetables, such as squash, eggplants, okra, cabbages, red and green peppers. Vegetable salads, etc. - Variety of fresh fruits and berries, fruit cups in natural juice. - Fresh starchy tubers such as potatoes, sweet potatoes, arrow roots, cassava, etc. - Buy whole grain foods such as maize, variety of beans, peas, lentils, rice, quinoa, whole grain chapatis etc. - Buy different types of fish, lean meats, such as chicken, lean goat meat, beef, and lean lamb meat etc. - Fats: vegetable oils, peanut and almond butter, avocados, butter in small amounts. Mustard, nuts, seeds and seed butters.	- Restrict items such as cake muffins (e.g., blueberry or corn muffins, croissants, breakfast biscuits, sweetened cereals, high fat breakfast sandwiches), coffee drinks such as frappuccinos, and high sugar lattes. - Bacon scrapple high fat breakfast sausages and Italian-style dinner sausages. Spare ribs and pork ribs. - Avoid frozen vegetables in butter sauce, high fat frozen meatballs, and spaghetti dishes. Alfredo sauce meals, pizza, frozen fried wings. - Fried potatoes / French fries, fried plantains, fried rice. - High calorie cookies, cakes and cupcakes, potato chips, candy bars, pies, ice cream etc. - Sodas, fruit flavored drinks, milkshakes, beers, wines, sweet drink mixes, and energy drinks. - Creamy salad dressings, lard, ghee.

Food Prepping for Weight Loss

Food prepping for weight. Food prepping is a process of planning meals and precutting foods ahead of time to allow quick healthy meal preparation throughout the week. Food prepping is an important step for people who are trying to eat healthy, but at times, are too busy or too tired due to long work hours, school, or busy with other daily activities. Busy parents, working college students, and those working long hours may get home too tired to start chopping onions, cutting vegetables and meats to make a meal, and might end up ordering fast foods or quick meals, such as roasted red meats, chapatis to go, pizza, fried chicken, french fries/chips, etc., as quick dinner meals. The problem with such quick meals is that the foods are usually high in fat, high in calories, and contribute to unwanted weight gain. Food prepping could help reduce intake of these high-fat foods.

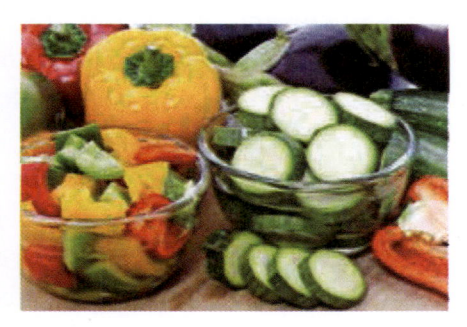

Food prepping includes washing, chopping or cutting different vegetables such as kale, cabbages, carrots, onions, etc., it also includes cutting and seasoning meats ahead of cooking time. Foods such as meats could be, seasoned, or marinated and stored, ready to cook. Seasoned meats could be stored frozen in one meal portions to be defrosted as needed for family meals. Meat should be thawed in refrigerator overnight for food safety. Cut-up vegetables stores well in clear covered containers or plastic storage bags. Use tight sealed bags or containers for aromatic items such as onions to prevent onion aroma in other fresh foods. Cut-up vegetables usually remain fresh in refrigerator for up to four days. Include at least two types of vegetables in family meals for variety. Vegetables are very low in calories, they make meals more colorful, and they increase fiber content of meals which promotes weight loss.

Cooking Methods

Food preparation methods have an effect in total calorie contents of meals. Foods that are deep fried contain more calories than baked, grilled, stir-fried, and steamed foods. Fats provide about 45 calories per teaspoon. Limiting amount of fats used in cooking foods results in reduced calories intake. A good example of how fat adds calories in diet is a comparison of fried potato vs baked potato. A medium-size baked potato provides about 150 calories, while medium-size deep fried potatoes yields about 400 calories. Baked or oven roasted chicken breast contains about 180 calories while a crispy fried chicken breast from the famous American KFC contains about 375 calories. The two examples, clearly shows how frying foods increases calories and sometimes almost doubles the calorie content of foods and leads to unwanted weight gain. For healthier low-calorie meals, choose stir-fried lean meats and vegetables meals, use grilled or baked foods, roasted meats, rotisserie chicken, instead of fried chicken. Make a large tray of oven-roasted mixed vegetables, tossed or brushed with small amount of vegetable oil and sprinkled with spices for a low-calorie side dish.

Portion Control

Healthy lifestyle changes for weight loss not only include healthy food choices but also healthy foods served in the right amounts or moderate portions. Healthy meals should be balanced in the three macronutrients, which are proteins, carbohydrates, and fats. The fats should be limited to small amounts of healthy fats, such as olive oil or canola used in cooking, and healthy low-calorie dressings used in vegetable salads. For protein foods, choose a variety of grilled or baked fish, such as salmon, tilapia, tuna, trout, etc. Choose lean meats, such as chicken and turkey or ground turkey instead of ground red meats. Include complex carbohydrates, such as whole grains, beans, and baked white or sweet potatoes, beans, steamed brown rice, or corn/maize. Include a variety of leafy green, cabbages broccoli, peppers, collards, vegetable salads etc. as the major part of your meals. Whole grains and vegetables are high in fiber are more filling and take longer to go through the gut.[62] Weight loss meals should contain larger portions of vegetables than meats and starch. Research shows that people get full by the amount of food they eat, not the number of calories they consume. Consuming the right

---

[62] Don Colbert, *I Can Do This Diet*, 68.

combination of foods provides the body with enough nutrients and fuel to remain energized but still continue to burn fat.

The recommended portions for weight loss is about 50 percent cooked vegetables about 25 percent lean meats and 25 percent starchy foods. Both proteins and fats take longer to digest and reduces feelings of hunger shortly after eating meals; the fiber in whole grains and vegetables adds bulk to the meals, which promotes feelings of fullness and helps reduce eating large portions than needed. Men have higher calorie and protein requirements than women and should consume slightly larger portions with each meal. Use medium-size plates instead of large plates for portion control. Take time to eat and enjoy your meals. Its takes about 20 minutes for the brain to send satiety or fullness signals to the gut. People who eat quickly or fast eaters who finish their meals in less than 10 minutes might end up consuming more food and more calories than needed. Another cause of consuming larger portions than we need is eating while preoccupied with watching movies, sports, games, or other media activities, which is referred to as "mindless eating," that leads to consumption of large portions of high-calorie snacks, such as potato chips, cookies, fried wings, high-sugar beverages or beers. To reduce intake of high-calorie snacks, create a healthy environment by changing snacks and beverages in the home. During sports event, prepare healthy snacks ahead of time. Select or serve healthy items, such as fresh-cut fruits, a large bowl of popcorn, a tray of fresh-cut vegetables with a yogurt dip or humus.

Beverages

Beverages are part of the diet and contribute to total calories consumed in a day. Whether the beverage consumed is 100 percent juice, or high sugar beverages such as soda, or fruit punch, they all add calories to the total daily intake. However, juice is natural and more nutritious than the high sugar beverages. Other hidden sources of calories are sweetened coffee and tea drinks such as lattes, mochas, frappuccinos, etc. Most of these beverages contain about 450–500 calories per serving. Wines and alcoholic, mixed drinks, also contribute to daily calorie intake. Calorie content in alcoholic drink mixes could range from about 150–600 calories per glass and contribute to undesired weight gain. The best beverage choice for weight loss is water or sparkling water, which adds no additional calories, and helps with weight loss and keeps the body well hydrated. Making change from sweet teas, coffee, juice, sodas, wines, etc. to drinking water and calorie free beverages could help reduce weight by about 2–4 pounds a month. Recommended water intake is about 64 fld oz/8 glasses or more daily. Drink more in hot weather or during high physical activity.

Heathy Choices when Eating Out

Meals consumed outside the home, either from restaurants or fast-food restaurants could be a source of extra calories in the diet. Healthy home cooked meals provide better option for weight loss than restaurant meals. However, both fast foods and restaurants offer some healthy food choices on their menus. Most of them provides nutrition information either on their website or on the menus. Whenever you eat in restaurants, select meals from healthy food options list on the menu. Select heathy food items such as grilled, baked, or oven roasted meats. Avoid fried meats and food items that are covered in rich butter sauces or creamy sauces. Beware of extra calories in the form of creams and butter added to restaurant mashed potatoes, food items made with alfredo sauce, fried rice, fried plantains etc. Select tasty lower calorie options such as baked potatoes or baked sweet potatoes with butter on the side to limit amount of fat added to your meals. Include a side salad or extra vegetables on the plate. Limit high fat, high sugar dessert items such as cakes, cake cookies, and puddings and choose lower calorie options such as a small bowl of frozen yogurt topped with fruits or a bowl of fruit salad.

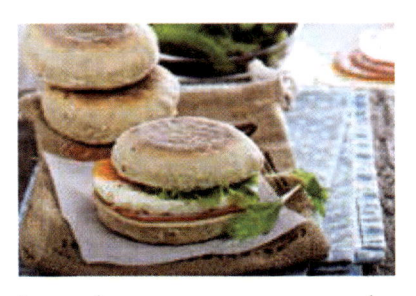

Exercise and Weight Control

Exercise is a great combination to healthy weight loss meals. Research shows that regular physical activity provides many health benefits including improved insulin sensitivity, controlled blood sugar, and decreased risk of type 2 diabetes, decreased risk of cardiovascular diseases, improved blood pressure, and decreased risk of colon and breast cancers.[63] Regular physical activity helps burn off calories and excess body fat. Include activities, such as riding a bike, playing different sports, walking on treadmill, dancing, working out in gyms, swimming, and taking a brisk walk in the trails, etc. All exercise provides health benefits and helps promote weight loss. People who work manual jobs such as warehouse workers, farm workers, and people in jobs that require lifting, pulling, hauling heavy items may require less exercise due to their level of physical activity during work hours. The World Health Organization's physical activity recommendation for adults is minimum of 150 minutes of moderate activities a week, or 30 minutes, five days a week. Exercise helps reduce body fat, builds lean muscle, strengthens bones and joints, and helps maintain healthy body weight. If you have not been exercising or you live a sedentary lifestyle, start with short walks, 10-minute walks or other exercises daily; increase exercise gradually and build to 20, 30, 45 minutes or more, five days a week.

---

[63] World Cancer Research Fund, 28.

Maintaining Weight Loss

Attaining your weight loss goal and maintaining the new or desired weight require focus and consistency of healthy lifestyle changes in regular physical activity and healthy food choices. Lifestyle change includes continuous meal planning and food prepping ahead of time to reduce days of unplanned high-calorie meals. It also requires consistency in selecting healthy low-calorie foods. Making healthy lifestyle changes results in sustainable weight-loss and well-maintained weight.

- Create a healthy food environment. Healthy food shopping helps change snacks in the home from high-calorie snacks, high in fat and sugar, to healthy snacks. Looking at a cake or cookies on your kitchen counter usually results in eating cake or cookies. It becomes a self-sabotage when you're trying to eat healthy. Create a healthy environment by replacing those high-calorie snacks with a tray of fresh fruits, popcorn, fruit cups, etc.
- Meal satisfaction: Avoid monotony in your meals. Boring diets are short-lived and cause people to return to unhealthy food habits. Making healthy low-calorie meals that are flavorful and tasty results in meal satisfaction with an outcome of successful weight loss.

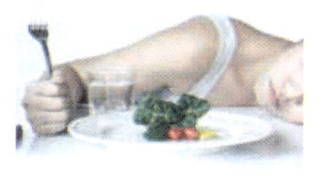

- Comfort foods: Emotional eating when feeling stressed or frustrated leads to weight gain. Overeating snacks that some people use as comfort foods, such as candy bars, potato chips, cookies or ice cream causes quick weight gain and more stress. To restrict high-calorie snacks, stock your kitchen pantry with healthy alternatives, such as popcorn, pretzels, and fruit cups. Place your favorite single-serving yogurts in the freezer to replace ice cream. Plan your snacks ahead of time.

Keep in mind, changing from high-fat meals and snacks to healthy lifestyles may take time, but it's the small steps of change that yields gradual permanent weight loss. The expected weight loss goal is four to five pounds every month. In six months, you would lose about twenty-five to thirty-five pounds or more of sustainable weight loss. Every fifteen to twenty pounds weight loss results in change of dress or pant size. As you continue to lose weight, celebrate your achievements. Give yourself nonfood rewards, such as a new dress or jewelry. Enjoy the journey to a new smaller heathier you.

CHAPTER 6

Lifestyle Change & Sample Menus

for Diabetes, Cancer, Heart Disease, & Weight Loss

According to research in psychology, change is a process that takes several steps. Making any behavior change could take more than twenty-one days to adjust to or get used to.[64] The steps of behavior change referred to as stages of change starts with contemplating or thinking about desired change, preparing for the change, followed by taking the action required to make change, and plans to maintaining the changes. Likewise, when making changes to a healthy lifestyle such as healthy food choices, starting an exercise regimen, or other change in behavior, it could take more than three or four weeks to adjust to. When initiating healthy lifestyle changes, give yourself time for gradual change.

---

[64] https://www.niddk.nih.gov/health-information/diet-nutrition/changing-habits-better-health.

The World Health Organization recommendations include regular physical activity and healthy diets as an ideal way to reduce the risk of chronic illnesses that have become prevalent in many nations. Most chronic illnesses are often related to unhealthy lifestyles such as smoking, sedentary lifestyles, and poor food choices. Following diagnosis of chronic illness such as hypertension, high cholesterol, or diabetes, healthcare providers usually recommend change of diet to healthier food choices, they may also recommend increased exercise to help control blood sugars, improve blood pressure, or blood cholesterol levels. They may also recommend that patient meet with a registered dietitian/nutritionist for guidance with food choices. When faced with chronic illness or other health concerns, it's important that we initiate recommended lifestyle changes. Research studies have proven that when people adopt to the Western diet, which is high in fat, high in meats but low in vegetables, and low in fiber, they become more susceptible to obesity illnesses such as diabetes, hypertension, and cardiovascular diseases.[65] It's important to evaluate our lifestyles, food habits, and make consistent healthy lifestyle changes for treatment and for prevention and treatment of chronic diseases.

Healthy Sample Menus

A positive change to healthy food choices and meal planning and increased physical activities promote the best outcomes for weight loss, prevention of chronic

---

[65] *Journal of Today Dietitian*, 21, no 2, 27.

illnesses, reversing high blood sugars, high-blood pressure, and blood cholesterol levels. Good nutrition helps restore body cells by providing them with vital nutrients, vitamins, minerals, and microminerals that are missing in most processed foods. Restored body cells give the body weapons to fight disease and restore healthy balance in the body. This chapter provides examples of basic healthy menus for weight loss and for chronic illnesses. The foods used in the sample menus could be replaced with other healthy choices based on the individual's taste, food likes and dislikes, or in case of food allergies. Table 2B in chapter 2 provides a list of options.

The first category of menus is on weight loss. The first recommendations for losing weight is to stop dieting and start a healthy lifestyle that includes eating healthy meals regularly, whether eating at home or in a restaurant. These sample weight-loss menus could be used as a template that guides you in making healthy selections of foods you like. Healthy food selection allows one to make low-calories, well-balanced meals with adequate balance of macronutrients and just enough calories to allow the body to burn off fat. The meals have to be healthy and tasty. To create tasty weight-loss meals, use cooking methods, such as grilled foods, oven-roasted and stir-fried foods. Home-cooked meals provide best options for healthy low-calorie weight-loss meals that are high in important nutrients. Buying a croissant which is a high fat, white flour pastry may contain about 250 calories or more but very low in nutrients compared to eating oatmeal topped with berries. A 300-calorie meal high in fiber which provides fullness and phytonutrients to keep you healthy. Healthy weight-loss meals should include whole grains and vegetables for high-fiber content. Vegetable can be easily added in all meals.

The Right Plate Mix

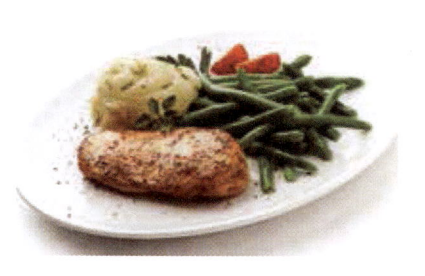

Recommendations for a healthy weight loss plate includes large servings of vegetables, moderate amounts of complex carbohydrates, and moderate portions of protein foods and carbohydrate foods. Include protein foods such as beans, lentils, and lean meats such as fish, chicken, turkey, and small amounts of red meats. Use complex carbohydrates such as steamed potatoes, sweet potatoes, or whole grains such as rice, noodles, maize/corn, and ugali in moderate amounts. Serve large portions of vegetables about 1/2 the plate, about 1/4 plate meats or beans, 1/4 plate starchy foods following the healthy plate guide. Fried foods should be limited due to their high calorie contents. Starchy foods, such as potatoes, sweet potatoes, and plantains, usually soak up a lot of oil during the frying process and could double the amounts of calories compared to baked or oven roasted. When eating out in restaurants, avoid high-calorie fried appetizers, foods such as fried wings, fried chicken strips, fried polenta, fried onion rings, etc., and replace such items with a small salad or cut vegetables with humus, grilled shrimp, grilled chicken lettuce wraps, etc. Order meals from the healthy menu items. Select healthy low-calorie beverages with meals.

Weight Loss Sample Menus:
Smaller portions are for women and large portions are for men.

Day	Breakfast	Lunch	Dinner	Snack
Day 1	1–2 egg omelet mixed with 1 slice of cheese, spinach onions, red peppers, garlic, etc., stir-fried with small amounts of olive oil. Serve on whole-grain toasts, 1–2 slices. Coffee or tea with low-fat creamer, either 1 pear, plum, or orange.	About 3–4 oz. sliced chicken sandwich on whole grain bread with mustard, lettuce, tomatoes, onions, etc. Small bowl of stir-fried cabbage. One fresh fruit of choice. Water	About 4 oz oven-roasted tilapia, 1–1.5 cup oven-roasted potatoes, a cup of stir-fried cabbage or broccoli, fresh fruit of choice, water.	One cup yogurt water

	Breakfast	Lunch	Dinner	Snack
Day 2	1–2 cup oatmeal, topped with cinnamon, blueberries, half a cup blue or blackberries, one small banana, coffee/tea (optional: 1 tsp. of sugar) or truvia, water	Large vegetable salad with lettuce or kale, tomatoes, cucumbers, red peppers, purple onions etc. light dressing, 3–4 oz grilled fish, your choice of fish such as tuna, whiting, trout etc., 1 small bowl of Fresh fruit and avocado salad, water.	Medium size bowl of Lentil and vegetable soup (onions, garlic, green and red peppers, 1–2 medium whole grain chapati 1 cup fresh fruit mix. Water	1/4 cup mixed nuts and water

	Breakfast	Lunch	Dinner	Snack
Day 3	1-2 English muffins (2 for men) with one to two teaspoons peanut butter, small bowl of diced mango or 1/2 of large mango, one yogurt, coffee/tea	About 4 oz chicken with one cup stir-fried carrots, peppers, garlic, onions, squash, broccoli served over 1–1.5 cup steamed rice. Water	Medium bowl of black beans stew with garlic and onions, large baked potato with ½ teaspoon butter, one cup stir-fried garlic spinach. Fresh fruit salad and water	Small bag of light popcorn, water

Note: For peanut allergies use regular butter in same amounts. Fresh fruits include one medium pear, apple, orange, small bananas, etc. One cup yogurt could be replaced with one cup of 2 percent milk.

Cancer-Fighting Foods

Plant foods have been proven to contain nutrients with powerful anticancer effects. According to the World Cancer Research Fund, plant foods provide the body with anti-inflammatory effects and nutrients proven to inhibit cancer cell growth. Since cancer cells tend to grow faster with high-body inflammation, we need to consume foods with the anti-inflammatory molecules as part of our regular diets. Vegetables, beans, fruits, whole grains, and nuts contain nutrients that are highly powerful in preventing cancer, destroying and removing cancerous cells out of the body. To the contrary, there's strong research evidence showing that red meats and processed meats are causes of colon and rectal cancers and are also associated with increased risk of cardiovascular diseases. Cancer-preventive diets should contain mostly plant proteins and small amounts of lean meats, such as chicken fish, eggs with no processed meats. This category of menus use mostly plant proteins, complex carbohydrates from whole grains, such as millet, oatmeal, and starchy tubers. The meals contain a variety of colorful vegetables of both cooked and salads, berries, citrus fruits, and nuts. Plant-based protein powders could be included as part of this diet. Add powder to fresh vegetables, such as cooked beets, baby kale, spinach, organic carrots etc., sweetened with fruit to make a smoothie. The spices included in these menus contain antioxidants and phytochemicals known to fight cancer cells and tumors as discussed in chapter 3. Cancer-fighting diets should include 6 or more servings of different varieties of colorful vegetables, 3–5 servings of berries, and citrus fruits as part of diet.

Cancer-Fighting Sample Menus: Consume your regular portions. If experiencing nausea from cancer treatment, consume small meals six times a day, eat cooked vegetables in place of salads, and peeled fruits.

Cancer-Fighting Sample Menus

Day	Breakfast	Lunch	Dinner	Snack
Day 1	1 Egg omelet made with (garlic, onions, red and green peppers, turmeric, and black pepper). Two slices whole grain toast with one teaspoon peanut butter. Unsweetened green tea, a small bowl of papaya cubes mixed with berries	Large salad (chopped kale, shredded purple cabbage, tomatoes, cucumbers peppers, ¼ cups almonds or mixed nuts), low-fat dressing and grilled chicken. One bowl of bean and maize/corn stew with potatoes, tomatoes, etc., fresh apple or pear, water.	Oven roasted tilapia or tuna fish, oven-roasted potatoes, large serving stir-fried cabbage with garlic turmeric, black pepper. Fresh orange or a small bow of papaya, water	Moringa shake: 1 banana, ½ cup pineapples, 2 tsp moringa powder, 1 cup coconut water or almond milk. Blend for 1–2 minutes to smooth consistency

	Breakfast	Lunch	Dinner	Snack
Day 2	Oatmeal or millet hot cereal with added cinnamon, two tablespoon raisins Bowl of mixed berries strawberries, blueberries and black berries topped with avocado. Hot green tea or regular black tea.	Small bowl cooked split peas stew, a plate of stir-fried mixed vegetables—carrots, peppers, garlic, onions, squash, broccoli—seasoned with garlic and turmeric. Served with sweet potatoes, fresh fruit, water	Lentil vegetable stew with carrots tomatoes, garlic red peppers. Served with whole grain chapati. Fresh fruit, water or green tea	Spinach avocado pineapple ginger smoothie. *Recipe: 1 cup baby spinach, 1 medium apple cut into cubes or (1 cup pineapple cubes,) 1 medium size banana, 1/8 avocado, ½ teaspoon grated ginger, 1 cup almond milk. Place apple and banana in blender, add spinach avocado and ginger, add almond milk and blend 1–2 minutes to smooth consistency*

	Breakfast	Lunch	Dinner	Snack
Day 3	A bowl of steamed-white potatoes and orange sweet potatoes diced and stir-fired with onions, garlic, ginger, cumin, turmeric, black pepper, and salt. 1 fresh cup yogurt, coffee/tea, Yogurt could be replaced with 1 cup milk, or 1 cup kefir	Black beans vegetable of choice stew. Use variety of vegetables. Serve with either steamed potatoes, cassava or yams. One bowl mixed berries, red, black, or blueberries, water	Grilled salmon with steamed brown rice, stir-fried broccoli and carrots. Fresh fruit of choice, water	One cup yogurt topped with mixed berries Water

Note: Drink 64 fld. oz or more water. Avoid sugar-sweetened beverages such as sodas and fruit punch etc. Snacks could be consumed at any time of the day.

Balanced Carbohydrate Meals for Diabetes Management

Diabetes and the health complications resulting from diabetes can be prevented through healthy-balanced meals and regular exercise. Reversing blood sugars to normal levels requires well-planned healthy meals. The key is balance in carbohydrate intake in each meal. The three carbohydrate food groups are starches, fruits, and milk (kefir/yogurt). These foods are needed in the body as the main source of energy and should be part of healthy meals but in controlled portions. Center for Disease Control recommends carbohydrate intake of three to four servings for women and about four to five servings per meal for those diagnosed with diabetes.[66]

Carbohydrate requirements change based on gender and activity level of individuals. Those working sedentary jobs need less carbohydrates than people who work in very active jobs. To plan healthy meals for diabetes, we need a good understanding of the carbohydrates/sugar contents of different foods and their serving sizes. One serving size in all food groups provides an equivalent of about 15 grams of carbohydrates. A good example of different serving size is berries versus grapes. Berries are lower in sugar, have a serving size of 1 cup compared to grapes, which are sweeter, and the serving size is 1/2 cup. When read-

---

[66] https://www.cdc.gov/diabetes/managing/eat-well/diabetes-and-carbohydrates.html

ing food labels, you might note the change in serving size of different foods, such as cereals, noodles, rice, etc.—change from 1 cup to 1/2 cup. The serving size of cooked oatmeal, mashed potatoes, and sweet potatoes is 1/2 cup, but serving size of cooked cassava, arrowroots, and rice is 1/3 cup. This means the foods with smaller serving sizes are higher in carbohydrates. Example: one cup of rice, one cup polenta, ugali, and cassava provides about 45 grams of carbohydrates; one cup of potatoes contains 30 grams of carbohydrates. Table 2B in chapter 2 provides more examples of different servings sizes. The menus in this category contains a range of four to five servings of carbohydrates. Women need three to four servings per meal, and men need four to five servings per meal. To lower carbohydrate amount in a meal by one serving, you could either reduce portions of starchy foods or avoid eating fruit with that meal.

Carbohydrate-Controlled Diabetes Menu:
Women need 3-4 servings; men need 4-5 servings.

Day	Breakfast	Lunch	Dinner	Snack
Day 1	One boiled egg, two turkey sausages, two slices whole grain toast with butter, a large banana, coffee / tea, water	Baked fish (whiting or tilapia), one cup cooked kale or collards, 1–1 1/2 cups ugali. One fresh fruit of choice and water	Oven-roasted chicken. 1–1 1/2 cup roasted sweet potatoes, stir-fried cabbage. One fresh fruit and water	One cup yogurt
	Breakfast	**Lunch**	**Dinner**	**Snack**
Day 2	1.5 cups oatmeal with one tablespoon raisins. One cup vanilla yogurt, 1/2 cup berries. Coffee/tea, water	1 cup black bean and carrot stew, 1 cup spinach. 1–1 1/2 cups mashed potatoes or steamed sweet potatoes, one fresh fruit, water	Roast beef, 1–1 1/2 cups mukimo, stir-fried cabbage. One fresh fruit, water	One slice toast with peanut butter, water

	Breakfast	Lunch	Dinner	Snack
Day 3	1/2–1 whole grain bagel with cream cheese or peanut butter, one fresh fruit of choice, coffee/tea	Stir-fried chicken, roasted chicken with one cup stir-fried vegetables—carrots, peppers, garlic, onions, squash, broccoli over 1 cup pilau rice, one fresh fruit water	Grilled salmon, 1–1 1/2 cups oven roasted potatoes or sweet potatoes, large serving of spinach with garlic and onions, one banana, water	1/4 cup mixed nuts and a small bowl of popcorn Water

Note: *Men need additional one to two servings of carbohydrates per meal.* Avoid sugar and sweetened beverages.

Note: Use fresh fruits to add flavor to smoothies and cereals. Whole grains are an important part of this meal plan. *Mukimo and ugali dishes could be replaced with same amounts of mashed potatoes, cassava sima, South African pap, phutu, phaleche, and West African yam or cassava fufu (approximately two to three servings of carbohydrates per cup).

Heart Health: Low Cholesterol Sample Menus

One of the major causes of heart disease is cholesterol build up in the arteries that surround the heart. A condition that puts the heart muscles at risk of reduced blood flow, reduced supply of oxygen and nutrients to the heart. Cholesterol buildup could block the arteries completely, causing a heart attack. It is highly important that we limit high-fat, high cholesterol foods known to cause arterial plaque buildup or atherosclerosis disease. Cholesterol and saturated fats are found only in animal foods. Eggs, shellfish, and high fat red meats contain higher amounts of cholesterol than lean meats. To prevent this deadly cholesterol buildup, we need to consume foods that lower blood cholesterol naturally. The meals should include high-fiber plant foods, such as beans, lentils, nuts, vegetables, fruits, which helps lower blood cholesterol levels. Diets high in fiber have been linked to reduce risk of heart diseases and stroke.[67] Plant foods, such as beans, nuts, broccoli cabbages, and spinach, contains vitamins that help the body make the antioxidant CoQ10 known to promote healthy heart and blood vessels. A heart-healthy diet also includes foods that help lower blood pressure. The diet should include foods high in whole grains, vegetables and fruits that are high in potassium, magnesium, and calcium minerals that have been proven through research to lower blood pressure in people with hypertension.

Heart-healthy meals should be prepared using healthy vegetables oils, such as canola, safflower oil,

---

[67] Bond Brill, 58.

olive oil, and other vegetable oils and limit uses of high-cholesterol animal fats, such as butter, lard, and ghee. The foods should be seasoned with spices to add flavor and to reduce the use of salt in cooking. Include heart-friendly omega 3 fatty fish, such as salmon, tuna, herring, mackerel, sardines, and lake Victoria's omena for flavorful meals. Season foods with herbs and spices, such as garlic, onions, cumin, ginger, black pepper, hot peppers, cinnamon, gloves, etc. The sample menus in this category contain foods that help lower blood cholesterol, foods that help lower blood pressure for those with hypertension without negative effects on people with healthy blood pressure.

Heart Healthy Menus

Day	Breakfast	Lunch	Dinner
Day 1	Lightly-steamed potatoes and orange sweet potatoes—diced and pan-fried with onions, garlic, ginger, cumin and black pepper. Pear or apple. A cup of hot cocoa or tea	Fish and vegetable stew served with brown rice, side salad with clear dressing, fresh fruit of choice, water	Oven roasted tilapia, oven roasted cut red potatoes, fresh vegetable medley (broccoli, cauliflower, red peppers) stir-fried with onions and garlic, water, fresh fruit
	Breakfast	**Lunch**	**Dinner**
Day 2	Bowl of oatmeal with 2% milk, topped with mixed berries. Cup of hot cocoa made with 1% or 2% fat milk, 1–2 teaspoons cocoa powder. A banana	Black beans with onions, ginger, tomatoes, and garlic, steamed brown rice, a bowl of spinach with onions and garlic, water	Baked chicken vegetable stir-fry using variety of mixed vegetables, steamed sweet potatoes, fresh fruit, water

	Breakfast	Lunch	Dinner
Day 3	Two slices whole grain toast with peanut butter, one cup low fat yogurt topped with berries, one apple, coffee or tea, water	Red beans and vegetable stew, served with whole grain chapati, a bowl of mixed fruit salad, water.	Baked salmon, ugali* and large servings of collard greens made with ginger onions and tomatoes. Mixed nuts (1/4 cup) and fresh fruit

Ugali could be replaced with mashed potatoes, yams, cassava, or West African fufu. Add snacks to these menus as needed. Use whole grains as corn chips with salsa or avocado dip, cut vegetables mixed with cut fresh fruits

Maintaining Heart Health

Prevention of heart disease requires continuous intake of grains, vegetables, and fruits that deliver high amounts of vitamins, minerals, soluble fiber, and antioxidants that naturally reduce LDL cholesterol that creates blockages in blood vessels. Plant foods provides the body with anti-inflammatory molecules which helps improve blood vessel health. Making change to a cholesterol-free, low-sodium diet is an important step toward improving heart health. Start substituting meats with beans three days a week, increase omega 3 fish in diet and reduce high fat red meats. Replace high cholesterol butter pastries with healthy snacks, such as berries, citrus fruits, nuts, and seeds. Every small change yield great health benefits.

CHAPTER 7

The Healing Kitchen: Using Superfoods to Fight Chronic Diseases

Superfoods are plant foods that have been proven through research to provide health benefits, such as disease prevention or aid healing in the body. Such foods are referred to as superfoods or functional foods. According to Harvard Medical School Health report, food is referred to as a superfood when it provides nutrients believed to offer health benefits beyond basic nutritional values. Foods are categorized as superfoods based on their content of disease-fighting nutrients such as vitamins, minerals, fiber, antioxidants, and phytochemicals that provides healing effects or improved health when consumed as part of a healthy diet. Examples of superfoods are oats, which contain the soluble fiber beta-glucan which is proven to lower LDL blood cholesterol, and the spice cinnamon, proven to help lower high blood sugars.[68]

---

[68] https://www.hsph.harvard.edu/nutritionsource/superfoods/

Healing foods have been used by our ancestors in every culture to treat family members from illnesses such as cough, common colds, and prevention of infection on skin cuts. Many of us have seen our parents or grandparents use certain foods such as honey and lemons for coughs and the common cold. They used ginger for nausea and upset stomachs. In our modern day, we know there are many other foods such as avocados, moringa leaves, beats and other foods that contain powerful healing properties but were not popular until recent years.

Growing up in the central region of Kenya, my siblings and I would visit our maternal grandparents during school breaks. Our grandparents lived on a small farm where they grew a variety of fruits, leafy green vegetables, and root tubers such cassava and yams. As young children, we spent most of the days playing in the farm, picking and eating sun-ripe juicy mangos, passion fruits, berries, and sugarcanes, but we never touched the ripe avocados that were falling off the trees. By lunchtime, we were too full to eat grandma's fresh boiled pumpkins and sweet potatoes and would have skipped dinner if our mom did not insist that we eat the mukimo meals. In recent years, avocado has become a popular healthy food item in many countries. It's used in homes and restaurants as cholesterol free fat used on toast instead of butter and added to deli, sandwiches in place of mayonnaise. Avocado is also used to top vegetables salads, used in health shakes, and in many other dishes. Pumpkins are also increasingly being used in recipes due to their high nutrient contents. In my recent visit to central Kenya, I noticed my family members were adding mashed pumpkins into chapati dough, giving the chapatis a soft texture and a beautiful hint of orange color.

About two years ago, I participated in a training seminar on healing foods which was offered by a medical doctor specialized in nutrition. The emphasis of this one-day seminar was on superfoods or foods that contained medicinal properties. Among the many foods discussed in this highly attended seminar, were foods such as coconut, green tea, and cocoa, and many other foods known to contain high amounts of powerful healing properties.[69] This chapter focuses on variety of plant foods and the different medicinal compounds in the foods, and the health benefits of consuming healthy diets combined with the superfoods. These superfoods are available in our very own farms, they are available in local farmers markets, and supermarkets.

Beets

Beets are highly nutritious great tasting vegetables used as a side dish or as one of the ingredients in vegetable salads. Beets are high in the minerals potassium and magnesium, known to help lower blood pressure. Beets also contain phytochemical that provide the body with bioactive molecules and

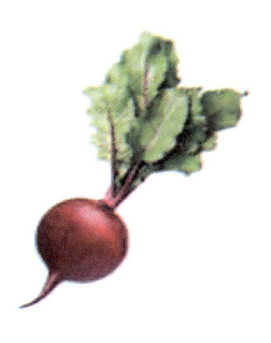

---

[69] Michael Lara, *Let Food Be Thy Medicine: A Practical Guide for Tapping into the Healing Power of Nutrients*, 50–53.

protects body cells from oxidative damage. The pigments that give beets their beautiful red-purplish color provides a powerhouse of detoxing and disease fighting molecules.[70]

- Beets provide detox power in the body. The phytochemicals in beets stimulate production of antioxidants in the liver, aiding the liver to detoxify itself and also remove toxins out of the body.
- Beets contain nitrates which helps relax blood vessels and helps lower blood pressure for people with hypertension.
- The leafy beet greens sometimes sold separately from the roots are packed with vitamin C, vitamin K, and folate, which are great for nourishing blood cells.

Recipes: Beet roots are commonly used in juicing recipes. Add fresh or cooked beets in fruit and vegetable shakes such as beet spinach and banana shake. Create beet juice recipes mixed with your favorite fruit. Cooked beet roots are also used in salads and soups recipes, and beet leaves make a tasty highly nutritious spinach-like side dish, either steamed or stir-fried.

---

[70] Joel Fuhrman, *100 Best Foods for Health and Longevity*, 25.

Broccoli

Broccoli belong in the cabbage group of vegetables referred to as cruciferous vegetables. Most people consume only the flowering top part of broccoli, but both the flower top and the soft part of the stalk are edible. Broccoli is easy to prepare and makes a tasty side dish. This highly nutritious vegetable provides a load of vitamin C, vitamin K, and several B vitamins. Broccoli also contains glucosinolates, powerful phytochemicals which provides body cells with anticancer activity, and a combination of antioxidants, anti-inflammatory and detoxification properties providing the body with powerful cancer-fighting effects.[71]

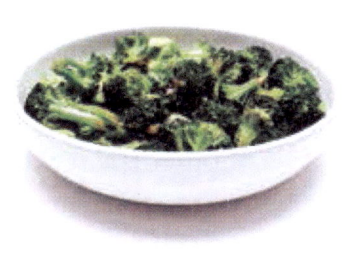

Cabbages

Cabbages contain minerals that are known to stimulate gastric juices for digestion and helps heal stomach and duodenal ulcers. Cabbages help stimulate production of glutathione in the liver, the body's natural antioxidant that helps with body detoxification and prevention of cell damage. The cabbage

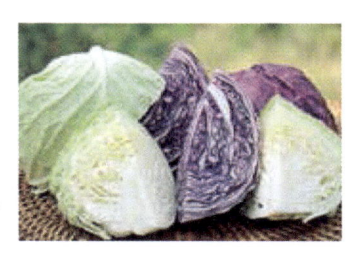

---

[71] Béliveau and Gingras, 88.

family—from the light green cabbage, the purple cabbage, to the crinkly dark green cabbage all contain compounds known to induce detoxification of carcinogens in the body, blocking tumor formation, and reducing the risk of developing cancer.[72]

- Brussels sprouts, also known as mini cabbages, provide similar nutrients and health benefits and contains higher amounts of anticancer molecules than the other cabbages.[73]
- Other leafy green vegetables containing large amounts of similar cancer-fighting compounds include kale, collard greens, and spinach.

Pumpkins

Pumpkin plants are farmed in most parts of Kenya and in many African countries. Pumpkin melons are commonly used as a side dishes, or added to stews to add flavor and color from its orange-yellow pigments. In United States pumpkins are used to add delicious flavors in coffees, sweet teas, pastries, cakes, pies and especially the very popular Thanksgiving Day pumpkin pie. Pumpkin melons have increased popularity in Kenya where it's used not only as a side dish but

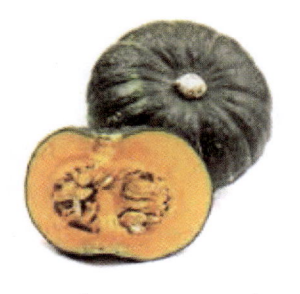

---

[72] Ramos, 52.
[73] DK Ramos page 52

also used as an ingredient in chapatis. Mashed pumpkin added to chapati dough gives chapatis a softer texture, and increases vitamins and mineral content while adding a nice hint of orange color to chapatis.

- Pumpkins are a low calorie and highly nutritious food. One cup of cooked pumpkin contains about 40 calories. It's loaded with the antioxidants lutein and beta-carotene and also high in vitamins A & E important for healthy eyes and silky smooth skin. Pumpkins are high in Vitamin C, and the important minerals iron, magnesium, potassium, and zinc.[74] The highly nutritious pumpkin leaves are commonly used as a side dish or added to potatoes, green bananas dishes, cassava dishes, and other dishes such as in mukimo dishes (a combination of bean corn/maize, potatoes, and leafy greens mashed together). When pumpkin leaves are mixed in with the rest of the ingredients in mukimo dishes, they add a light green color, great flavor, and most importantly, adds a load of vitamins and minerals to the dish.

Pumpkins seeds are good source of the healthy omega-3 fats and vitamins A, E, K, zinc, and iron. Pumpkin seed oils are known to improve men's health. The high content of the powerful antioxidant lycopene and the minerals zinc, iron, and selenium makes pump-

---

[74] Fuhrman, 100.

kin seed extracts a common over-the-counter supplement for prostate health, sold in many pharmacies as "pumpkin seed complex." Pumpkins seeds and pumpkin leaves are high in the mineral zinc that helps improve immune system and helps with healing of skin cuts and wounds.

Stinging Nettles

Stinging nettles have been used in many cultural meals for generations, but to the younger generations they might be a little intimidating as touching nettle leaves results in painful stings. Wear gloves to harvest and wash nettles to prevent stings. Once stir-fried or steamed, this wonderful vegetable has a delicious taste. Nettles have been used in many countries as natural cures for muscle and joint pains, arthritis, and gout as it helps remove uric acid from joints.[75] Nettles are also good sources of iron and vitamin C. Since iron is absorbed better in the gut when combined with vitamin C. The iron in nettles is more easily absorbed in the body.[76]

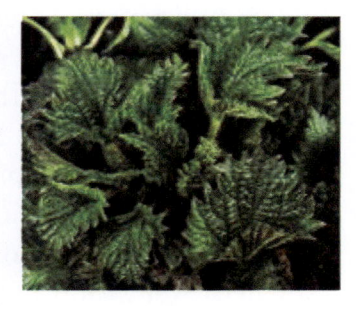

---

[75] Andrew Chevallier, *Herbal Remedies Handbook: Remedied for More Than 50 Common Conditions*, 234.
[76] Ramos, 72.

Moringa leaves, Pods and Seeds

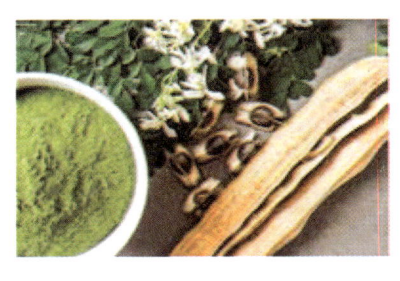

Moringa tree is often called the miracle tree. This name is befitting moringa due to its high nutrient content and multiple health benefits. Moringa trees are known to have originated from India but moringa trees grow and flourish well in many African countries and is commonly used by the people of Ghana and other West African countries. Moringa trees are draught resistant and do well in tropical and subtropical weather. In Eastern Africa, moringa is grown by farmers in many parts of Kenya but more heavily used by families in Northern Kenya mostly in Marsabit County, Southern Ethiopia, Sudan, and parts of Somalia and many other African countries.

In recent years, moringa has earned a new name among East Africans who call it "siri ya uchungu," or the secret of pain. There are many research articles and reports on health benefits of moringa tree contents of phytochemicals, and antioxidants that fight multiple illnesses.[77] Moringa trees yield edible leaves, pods, seeds, and flowers. The leaves and seeds are high in

---

[77] National Research Council. 2006. *Lost Crops of Africa: Volume II: Vegetables*. Washington, DC: The National Academies Press. doi: 10.17226/11763, https://www.nap.edu/read/11763/chapter/16#248.

protein and contains all essential amino acids. Moringa leaves also contain high amounts of iron, loads of vitamin C, vitamin A, important B vitamins, and minerals,[78] making moringa a highly valuable plant food that is nutritionally beneficial to all populations. Moringa is especially beneficial to people who live in dry parts of sub-Saharan African countries where children and families experience food insecurity during dry weather seasons. Other powerful health benefits of moringa include the following:

- High contents of polyphenols, and antioxidants known to fight cancer. Moringa helps fight cancer in many ways. It's known to reduce body inflammation which is a cause for cancer and other chronic illnesses. It reduces cancer cell proliferation and induces cancer cell death by apoptosis and removal of cancerous cells out of the body without damaging healthy cells.[79]
- Moringa has high contents of vitamin C, vitamin E, and the minerals calcium, magnesium, potassium, and zinc, nutrients known to help lower blood pressure. The high vitamin C and zinc contents helps promote healing of wounds and skin cuts.

---

[78]

[79] National Research Council. 2006. *Lost Crops of Africa: Volume II: Vegetables*. Washington, DC: The National Academies Press. doi: 10.17226/11763, https://www.nap.edu/read/11763/chapter/16#248.

- Moringa helps lower high blood sugar levels by reducing insulin resistance in the body.
- It also lowers blood cholesterol by lowering LDL levels in the blood. Moringa has several other health benefits.

There are several ways to use and benefit from this highly nutritious miracle tree. Freshly picked moringa leaves are prepared like collard greens or spinach and used as a side dish with ugali, pap or phutu meals in place of collard greens or kale. Dry moringa leaves are crushed and used to make moringa tea drinks or processed into a powder that is used in health shakes, added to soup, stews, or mukimo dishes.

Young long moringa pods are more like french green beans and could be diced up and steamed or stir-fried for use as a side dish or added to stews. Tender green moringa seeds harvested out of the ponds before they are dry are cooked in meals just like green peas. Dry seeds are mostly used for moringa oil, which is great for reducing body inflammation. No matter how you choose to eat moringa, whether you eat cooked moringa leaves, pods, or powder, moringa tree products provide protein, amino acids, iron, vitamins, and minerals in the diet, plus high amounts of phytonutrients with multiple health benefits.[80]

---

[80] https://www.researchgate.net/publication/323717202_Nutraceutical_or_Pharmacological_Potential_of_Moringa_oleifera_Lam.

Beans and Lentils

Beans and lentils are staple foods in African countries. Both are regularly used in many boarding school meals as a low-cost protein food. Bean recipes change slightly from culture to culture but they are basically consumed in all three meals of the day. Breakfast meals may include a bowl of beans and maize mix commonly called githeri in Kenya, a bowl of coconut flavored beans with bread, or beans with cassava etc. For lunch and dinner, many varieties of beans and lentils stews are served with complex carbohydrates such as rice, chapatis and ugali, bananas, or cooked combined as the popular rice and bean meals. Beans are highly nutritious foods and provides the macronutrients protein and carbohydrates and very small amounts of healthy fat. Beans also provide various essential B vitamins, the essential mineral iron, and disease-fighting antioxidants.[81] Beans are high in both soluble and insoluble fibers. Insoluble fibers provide benefits of maintaining gut motility, preventing constipation, and in maintaining a healthy colon. Beans are also high in soluble fiber, which helps control cholesterol levels in the blood by removing LDL cholesterol or bad cholesterol out of blood vessels. Beans are

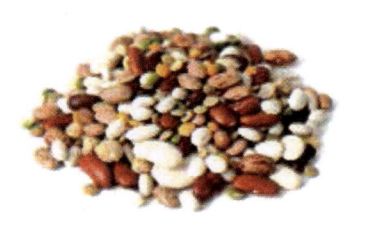

---

[81] Bond Brill, 114.

also high in potassium, magnesium, and microminerals good for regulating blood pressure.[82]

Millet

Millet flour is used to make one of the most popular fermented hot breakfast cereals in Kenya, Nigeria, South Africa, and many other African countries. Millet is also used to make breads and other dishes using mix of millet and maize flour which is more nutrient to meals such as millet ugali or millet pap. Millet is a staple food in African countries, Asia, and some European countries. In US, millet is increasingly being used as a gluten-free hot breakfast cereal that is nutritious and easy on the gut for people with gluten sensitivity. Millet contains B vitamins, magnesium, and is high in soluble fiber. The fiber in millet has been proven through research to significantly lower levels of triglycerides and lower LDL cholesterol while increasing HDL/good cholesterol and therefore a heart healthy food.[83] Millet also contains amino acids and the minerals iron, niacin, manganese, phosphorus, and potassium.

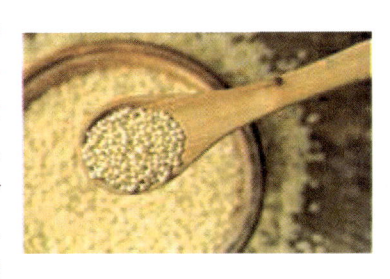

---

[82] Bond Brill, 115.

[83] https://wholegrainscouncil.org/whole-grains-101/whole-grains-101-orphan-pages-found/health-benefits-millet

Oatmeal

Oatmeal is a popular breakfast cereal in many parts of the world. Cooked oatmeal in a tasty nutritious cereal with the consistency of porridge. Oats contain beta-glucan a soluble fiber that transforms into a gel-like sponge in the gut that is excellent in removing LDL cholesterol out of the body, reducing the risk of heart disease.[84]

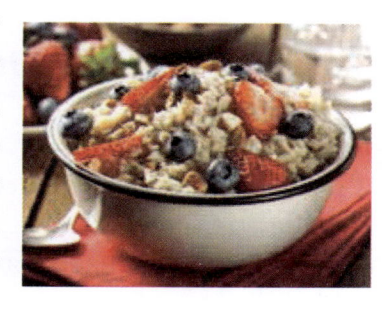

- Due to the high fiber content in oatmeal, it's digested slowly and moves through the gut at a slower pace, and helps control blood sugar for people with diabetes.
- Beta-glucan in oatmeal quickly lowers LDL or bad cholesterol in the blood. Consuming oatmeal for breakfast combined with healthy meals for lunch and dinner, reduces the risk of coronary artery disease.
- Oats are used in cold cereal, and as granola which is mostly used to top yogurt and fruit salads and as granola snack bars. Oatmeal is increasingly being used in diaspora by people from many parts of Africa not just as a breakfast cereal but also added to ugali, to cassava,

---

[84] Bond Brill, 61.

or yam flour to make a more nutritious fufu, a common dish among West Africans.

Super Nutrient in Fruits

Berries

All varieties of berries contain high amounts of nutrients with great health benefits. From wild-picked berries to farm-grown berries, such as golden berries, blackberries, strawberries, blueberries, raspberries, and mulberries, they all contain high amounts of vitamin C, vitamin A, potassium, magnesium, fiber, antioxidants, and phytonutrients with powerful anticancer effects. Blueberries contain nutrients that fight cancer cell proliferation and growth. Blackberries contain high amounts of antioxidants with detoxifying effects in the body. They also contain phytonutrients with anti-inflammatory and anticancer effects.[85]

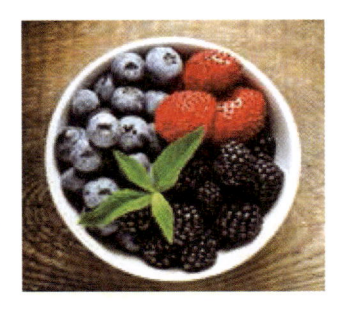

Apple

Apples grow well and are commonly consumed fruits in South Africa. Kenyan farmers are increasingly growing apple trees in the cooler parts of the country such as Nyeri, Kiambu highlands, Nandi hills, and Kitale and other areas in the country. Apples are

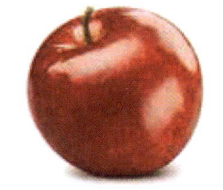

---

[85] Fuhrman, 27.

not only good as cash crop, but the health benefits of apples is good reasons for farmers to plant 1-2 trees where weather allows growth.

Apples are delicious low-calorie, sweet crunchy fruits that make a great snack any time of the day. Apples contain super nutrients with great health benefits, making the famous quote "An apple a day will keep the doctor away" true in many ways.

- Apples contain high amounts of vitamins and minerals, and antioxidants known to inhibit growth of cancerous tumors.[86] Phytonutrients in apples helps reduce body inflammation and helps with body detoxification. Apple skins contain both soluble and insoluble fiber known to lower LDL or bad cholesterol in the blood, reducing atherosclerosis disease which helps improve heart health. Wash apple skins well to remove any pesticides.

Cooking with Herbs and Spices

Cinnamon

Cinnamon is one of the most common spices among people of Eastern Africa. It is used to flavor tea, mandazi (a breakfast pastry), and used in rice pilau recipes, soups, bread and other foods. Cinnamon, cloves, and cardamons are highly nutritious spices used in many recipes by people residing in coastal regions of Eastern

---

[86] Fuhrman, 11.

Africa. The latest research on health benefits of cinnamon shows that this flavor-enhancing spice high in antioxidants has powerful effects in lowering blood sugar levels after meals and lowering blood triglyceride levels.[87]

Cinnamon contains phytochemicals proven to effectively reduce insulin resistance and lower blood sugar. The best quality cinnamon is Ceylon, also known as "true cinnamon." Use cinnamon in tea for added flavor, sprinkle cinnamon on buttered toast, or add to hot cereals such as oatmeal or millet. Cinnamon could also be added as a seasoning for beef and vegetable stew, in pilau recipes, or added to chapati dough for improved blood sugar control.

Cocoa

It is cultivated in many tropical countries in Western Africa and South America. Cocoa has been proven through many research studies to provide several health benefits. Health benefits of cocoa includes lowering blood pressure to normal levels without having negative effect on those with normal blood pressure. Cocoa contains phytonutrients and antioxidants that helps improve insulin sensitivity and lowers blood sugar levels for people with type 2 diabetes. Cocoa has also been proven to provides an anti-inflammatory effect for people suffer-

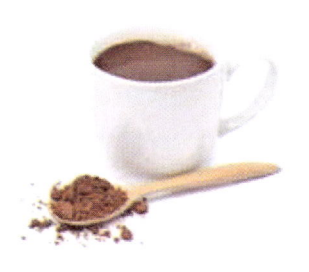

---

[87] Ramos, 116.

ing from diseases such as asthma or bronchitis.[88] Pure cocoa powder is not the same as hot chocolate or the high sugar chocolate candy bars. For the most health benefits of cocoa use pure cocoa powder. Add one tablespoon of pure cocoa powder in hot water or hot milk for a delicious beverage two times a day. Cocoa helps lower blood pressure, supports healthy artery functions and improves heart health.[89]

Garlic

Garlic is in the onion family and is one of the most commonly used spices in the world. It has been used in cooking since the days of the philosopher Hippocrates. Garlic not only adds great flavor to foods, but this spice has been proven to have many health benefits. Garlic promotes a healthy immune system, improved heart health, and contains cancer fighting compounds. Garlic provides powerful benefits on heart health by naturally lowering the unhealthy cholesterol (LDL) in the blood and preventing cholesterol buildup known to cause clogged up arteries.[90] By lowering LDL cholesterol buildup, garlic reduces atherosclerosis or hardening of arteries. Garlic also contains the compound sulfur known to help relax and improve elasticity of blood vessels, which helps lower blood pressure.

Garlic contains compounds that have cancer-fighting effects and is linked to reduced risk of colorectal,

---

[88] Lara, 50.
[89] Lara, 51.
[90] Ramos, 116.

breast, and prostate.[91] Garlic also contains phytochemicals known to play an important role in preventing cancers of stomach and colon. Choose fresh rather than jarred garlic for maximum health benefits. Garlic could be added to most dishes as desired from egg omelets, to vegetables stir-fry's, bean meals, Githeri meals, soups, stews, pilau dishes and could be used raw in salads, added to humus and avocado dips etc. Chopping or grating garlic and letting it sit for about 10–15 minutes before cooking helps boost availability of the healthy compounds in garlic.

Ginger

Ginger is used as tea mix commonly referred to in Eastern Africa as masala tea used in hot chai tea and as a cold beverage in ginger iced tea. Ginger is one of the most versatile roots used in many parts of the world as home remedy for nausea, upset stomachs, and motion sickness. The spice is also commonly used by pregnant women to reduce morning sickness. The active molecules in ginger called gingerol have anti-inflammation effects in the body and naturally relieves arthritic pain and reduces menstrual pains.[92]

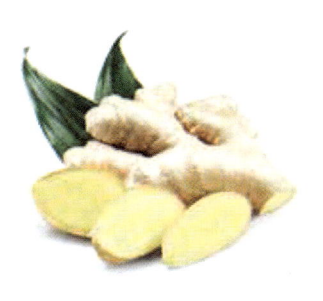

---

[91] Ramos, 116.
[92] Fuhrman, 58.

- Whenever possible, use fresh ginger instead of dry. Fresh ginger contains higher amounts of nutrients than processed.
- Ginger is also used in home remedies for the common cold and sore throat. Drink a cup of ginger tea with added honey and lemon.

Turmeric

Turmeric spice is known to have been used in ancient India dating far back to 500 BC.[93] Turmeric has remained a common ingredient in Indian and Middle Eastern recipes. In the modern day, turmeric is used in many other countries, especially the Caribbean islands and many African countries. In Kenya, turmeric is more heavily used by Kenyan Indians and by people in the coastal regions of East Africa and used less often by other communities.

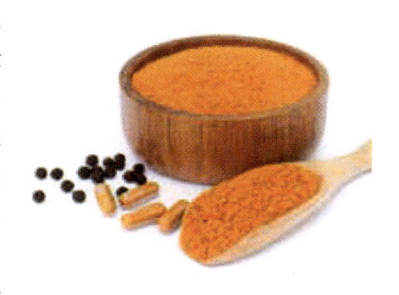

Turmeric contains the active compound curcumin, which gives the spice its vibrant yellow-orange pigments and powerful health benefits. You might find the terms *turmeric* and *curcumin* frequently used interchangeably. Curcumin has been proven through research to stop growth of cancer cells; it helps eliminate cancerous cells in the body through cell apoptosis without harming healthy cells.[94] Curcumin is also known for its mild

---

[93] Fuhrman, 58.
[94] Lara, 48.

anti-depressant effects. It also has anti-Alzheimer's effects through inhibiting the formation of abnormal proteins found in people suffering from Alzheimer's.[95]

Studies have also shown curcumin to contain anti-inflammatory properties known to reduce inflammation associated with arthritis and can be used to provide relief from rheumatoid arthritis. Curcumin is not easily absorbed in the body, but adding a pinch of black pepper to the spice enhances its absorption in the gut and makes it more effective.[96] This wonderful spice is tasty in meat curries, bean and lentil stews vegetables, stir-fried vegetables.

Healthy Fats

Avocados

Avocado fruit is known for its high content in vitamin E, and plant hormones that help lubricate joints and reduce arthritis symptoms. Several studies show that eating avocados decreases total cholesterol, LDL, and triglycerides and promotes healthy blood lipids.[97] Vitamin E in Avocado helps restore skin health and vitality. Vitamin E is known to many as the beauty or antiaging vitamin.

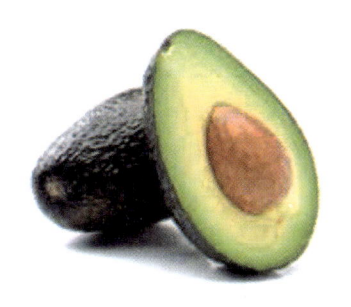

---

[95] Lara, 48.
[96] Lara, 51.
[97] Fuhrman, 16.

Avocado is also rich in glutathione, an important antioxidant in the body. Glutathione strengthens body cells, boosts the body's immune system, and helps the body fight infections and diseases.[98]

- One medium size avocado fruit contains about 4 grams of protein, but provides the equivalent of 5 teaspoons of fat/oil. Watch portions to prevent undesired weight gain.
- A medium-size avocado fruit provides ten to eleven grams of fiber, which is more than half of an adult's daily fiber requirements, great for prevention of constipation.
- Avocado is high in vitamin E and lutein, good for healthy skin, healthy joints, and eye health. Avocados provide cholesterol free healthy fats good for the heart.

Avocados could be added to a variety of dishes. They add great flavor to cooked rice, and could be easily added to dishes, and chapati vegetable roll-ups or use in Uganda's chapati vegetable and egg roll-ups referred to as *Rolex* in the streets of Kampala. Avocados taste great added to vegetable salads, fruit salads, smoothies and make a healthy alternative on toast instead of butter. Avocados are smooth textured fruits that add taste to baby foods. Use small portions, about ¼ of medium avocado mashed or mixed with other foods such as mashed

---

[98] Ramos, 50.

potatoes, peas, carrots, bananas to boost nutrients and flavor in baby foods.

Coconut

Coconut is an amazing fruit with nut-like shell. It is highly used in the Pacific region where it's referred to as the tree of life due to the various uses of coconut fruit. It provides coconut oil and coconut milk; coconut water and it's also used in skin care products. Coconut trees do well in hot humid coastal regions. Young green coconut fruits provide cool thirst-quenching water high in electrolytes, perfect for hot tropical weather. The mature inner flesh of coconut is usually grated and used as coconut milk, which is used in different recipes. Coconut milk is used in rice pilau, different types of vegetable and bean stews, and bean recipes such as breakfast beans/bahaazi mahamri. Coconut is loaded with super nutrients; antioxidants, vitamins, minerals, fiber, and a unique type of healthy fat which is referred to as MCT or medium chain triglycerides.[99] Coconuts provide the following health benefits:

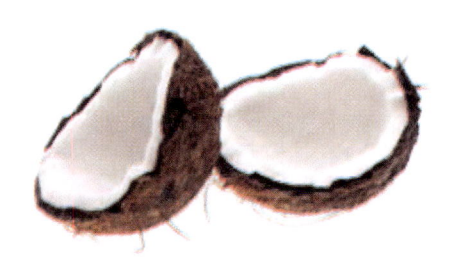

- Healthy fat in the form of MCT oil, which is proven to increase healthy cholesterol HDL

---

[99] Lara, 59.

without raising levels of LDL bad cholesterol, lowering the risk of heart disease
- Coconuts unique MCT fats can be used as alternative energy source of brain food, which is beneficial to people with Alzheimer's.[100]
- Coconut contains antiviral and antibiotic properties; Fats in coconut helps the body fight viruses that cause common colds and flu and helps the body combat bacteria that causes gum disease and urinary tract infections.

Nuts

Nuts provided the body with cholesterol-free fats, protein, fiber, and loads of vitamin E, which supports heart health and great for skin health. Nuts are also great sources of the minerals iron, zinc, folate, calcium and magnesium. Nuts provide the body with monounsaturated omega-3 fats known to lower levels of LDL cholesterol, keeps the arteries healthy, and improves heart health.[101] Eat a variety of nuts, such as walnuts, cashews, almonds, macadamia nuts, pistachios, etc. Limit potions to about 1/4 cup servings. Nuts are high in healthy fats, and large portions could cause unwanted weight gain.

Chapter Summary

This chapter on healing foods covers a small number of very important superfoods, and the numerous

---

[100] Ibid, 46
[101] Ramos, 92.

medicinal properties found in various plant foods. However, there are many to plant foods in different countries that have not yet been studied for their phytonutrient contents. Food science research regarding plant-food nutrition and the various health benefits of superfoods is ongoing and is updated continuously. Every chapter in this book highlights the importance of increasing consumption of plant foods in our diets for improved health. Plant foods fuel the body cells with healing phytonutrients and molecules that aid the body's biological processes of repair and healing. Continuously feeding the body with essential vitamins and minerals plays a major role in restoring body cells to health. It's important that we create healing kitchens in our homes by removing unhealthy food items referred to as "empty-calorie foods" or foods that provides calories from fats and sugar, causing weight gain and obesity, that are very low in vitamins and minerals. Change your food choices to whole grains, vegetables, fruits, beans, nuts, and small amounts of lean meats. A healthy meal pattern is not only important for maintaining healthy body weight but also vital for prevention of chronic diseases that bring havoc to families and communities. Healthy diets and healthy lifestyles are highly recommended in every home, in boarding schools and other academic institutions, and in public health and government institutions as key to improved health and well-being of individuals, families, and communities.

Eat to good health. Let food be your medicine.

ABOUT THE AUTHOR

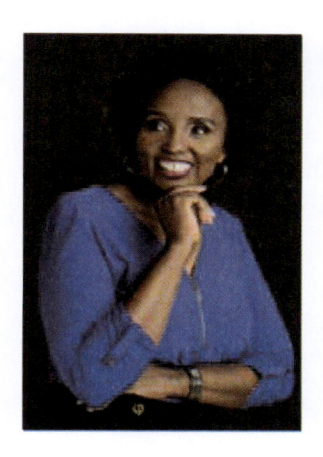

Rosemary is a Registered Dietitian, Certified Diabetes Care Specialist and Certified Healthy Lifestyle Coach in Maryland. She studied nutrition science at Montclair University in New Jersey and Morgan State University in Maryland. Rosemary has a graduate certificate in Business from John Hopkins University School of Business in Baltimore Maryland. Rosemary has been privileged to provide nutrition counseling and healthy lifestyles coaching in group settings, and to hundreds of individuals in the State of Maryland, Washington DC and Virginia areas. While Rosemary is specialized is diabetes prevention, and diabetes management, she also completely embraces the approach of using healthy diets as the first line of defense in prevention of chronic illnesses.

Rosemary has worked as a Nutritionist for Baltimore City Department of Health, in the Women Infant and Children's (W.I.C.) Program for over 12 years where she promoted healthy food choices and healthy lifestyle change for improved maternal health, improved pregnancy outcomes and the health of infants and children. She has worked as a Registered Dietitian/Nutritionist for over 20 years in various settings including hospitals and outpatient clinics and helped many individuals improve their health through change to healthy diets.

Due to her love of helping others improve their health through nutrition, Rosemary founded Affya Health and Wellness Center in Owings Mills Maryland. A company that uses the approach of healthy diets and lifestyle change to promote health and wellbeing in the local communities and surrounding areas.